June 1985

Happy Birthday!
Lots of Love,
Lisa & the Crew

Please Doctor, I'd Rather Do It Myself... with Herbs!

LaDean Griffin

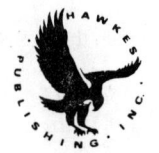

Published by
HAWKES PUBLISHING, INC.
3775 South 500 West
Salt Lake City, Utah 84115
Tel. (801) 262-5555

©1979
by LaDean Griffin
Salt Lake City, Utah

ISBN 0-89036-058-8

POEMS IN THIS BOOK BY NORENE HALLIDAY

Printed in the U.S.A.

Illustrations & Cover by
Rod Warren

TABLE OF CONTENTS

Physiology 1
   The Cycle.. 2
   Arteriosclerosis 5
   The Exocrine Glands 5
   The Symptoms 6
   Medical Treatments 6
   Narcotic Alkaloid 7
   Probable Cause 7
   Lady Slipper 8

Drugs.. 9
   Belladonna 9
   Chloral Hydrate 10
   Morphine 10
   Pentobarbital... 11
   Phenobarbital 11
   Secobarbital 12

Herbs... 14
   Vitamin A 19
   Vitamin B1 19
   Vitamin B2 19
   Vitamin B6 19
   Vitamin B12 20
   Vitamin C 20
   Vitamin D 20
   Vitamin E 21
   Minerals 21
      Calcium 21
      Iodine 21
      Iron... 21
      Magnesium 21
      Phosphorus... 21
      Potassium 22
   Herbs for Parasites 22
      Bacteria 23
      Salmonella 23
      Trichinosis 23
   Alfalfa for Everyone 25
      Arthritis 26
      Hormones 27

Ginseng for the Man 30
Golden Seal for the Diabetic 33
    Diabetes and Insulin 35
    Other Uses for Golden Seal 38
Kelp for Glandular Balance 39
Licorice for Hypoglycemia 42
Lobelia for Restoring the Sick 47
Saffron for Digestion and Stiffness 50
    Medical Research 51
    Why Saffron Helps 52
Yucca for Arthritis 53
    Yucca Extracts 53
Condiment Herbs 56
    Interesting Facts 57
    Vegetable and their Compatible Herbs & Spices 59
Cosmetic Herbs 61
    Suntanning 65
Nervine Herbs 65

Practice 70
    Modern-day Example 72

Conclusion 76
    The way to treat a Cold 81
    Recommended Reading 83

Physiology

WHEN we consider the dietary deterioration that is happening to most of the younger generation we might look at the kinds of foods young people live on from day to day — hamburgers, hot dogs, malts and candy bars. The school hallways display candy machines and most of the hot lunches are a poor substitute for the good nutritious mineral and vitamin-rich foods children need for proper growth and health. If we were going to build a beautiful home, we would not be interested in using faulty material. We would not build our home in such a way that it would collapse in a few weeks, yet when it comes to building beautiful, healthy bodies that have to last a lifetime, some parents give little regard to what their children eat.

Christ called the body a temple. Would we — should we — build this temple of rubbish and trash? Picture, if you can, the temple of life: A structure with four main pillars, where, if any one of the four is weak, that side could fall. Let us call each of these pillars of life by name because each plays an important part in the whole structure. One we will call the physical part, another the mental, the third the spiritual, and the fourth would certainly be the social. All of these parts, equally balanced, could maintain the roof, keeping us sheltered, peaceful, and secure. When any one of these areas is out of balance, on the total building, man's temple of life is affected. In order for one to be successful and have total health, all of these attributes must be fully active and functioning in his life. Often the first breakdown of the body will so affect us that discouragement, dejection, fear, and pain will leave no place for mental activity, social, or spiritual life, and leads to a one-sided person who is a drag on everyone around him. First and foremost we must keep the body well and functioning so that all other important parts of life can be enjoyed. Some people live so far out of their bodies doing all the social things, that they never give a thought to fuel until they run out of gas. Then others live so far out of this world, waiting for the next life spiritually, that they do not take care of the temple that they have been given to treasure and care for. There are still others, like the absent-minded professor, who never remembers to eat because he is too busy learning until he falls off his chair, and suddenly realizes "Oh, I'd better eat something."

Nothing lives unto itself alone. Where there are limitations of an organic nature, injury, or chronic congestion, the spirit within can find the route to liberation from such pain and disorder if such liberation is sought after. No matter how the body may be limited, the powers within can somehow find a way to maintain life.

THE CYCLE

Life is a song, a rhythm of harmony or discord and most of the time we rise and fall from one to the other. Recent studies show that we go through three cycles monthly — physical 23 days, emotional 28 days, and intellectual 33 days, each overlapping the other. If there were a physician who claimed he could bring the patient's body into perfect balance, he would only be kidding himself as well as his patient.

Sometimes all the imperfection around us, such as disease, broken bodies, and torn spirits, makes it difficult to understand why a just God would allow such disharmony. As we struggle with biorhythms and mental, physical, social, and spiritual levels of existence, it is often with difficulty that we maintain enough courage to seek answers to our health problems. The answers are there if we seek them. The reasons we have such problems may be made known to us also.

Who can tell his soul, "Peace be still," when all fury rages around and in him? Only he who has some sort of faith — faith in something, someone, some place, or some how. Only he who has hope for the future and courage for the day. All others will drop by the wayside, exhausted by the constant struggle that life presents.

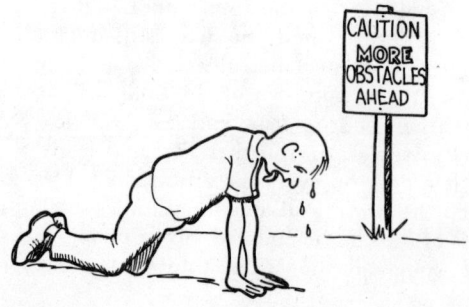

What is faith? Faith is the evidence of things hoped for within the scope of reality. There are some people who believe if they think about something long enough and hard enough they can think their way into or out of anything — changing anything. Such unrealistic faith would change even the way the sun comes up if it were possible. Positive thought and faith lead us along only on laws which already exist. If a person were born with half a brain, he could not think his way to brilliance. If he were born with only one leg or had one cut off, he could not think his way into a new leg.

We all have a built-in desire for perfection. We endlessly seek perfection around us. We have a tendency to look around us and note, "He's too skinny," or "He's too fat." Someone else may appear too small or too large, too this or too that. Critically we eternally search for perfection in others. Once in a while when we see someone we might feel is perfectly beautiful, we express such wonder to another person, who may promptly say, "Her? she isn't beautiful. Her nose is too long, or her eyes are too close together." Momentarily our idea of beauty is shattered.

Beauty is in the eyes of the beholder, but when we look at the whole person as a child of God we can find all kinds of perfection. When we live so as to see the spirit within and the aura without, we will then behold a beauty beyond all superficiality. Where there is beauty within ourselves, we will respond to such beauty in others.

In bio-rhythms, perfect balance is achieved only rarely and for short periods, as also a completely negative bio-pattern seldom occurs. The rest of the time it is up to the mind or the spirit (whatever you may choose to call it) to maintain its sanity balance in the center of the ebb and flow of life forces, both internal and external.

Man needs the full spectrum of natural light for all physiological functions, just as he needs full nourishment. The eyes need to be exposed to natural outdoor light. This light can be just as helpful in the shade, because when light strikes the eye's retina, all physiological functions of the body are stimulated. To be outdoors — but not necessarily in the sun — as many hours a day as possible improves general health. We know that sunshine has a definite improving effect on the endocrine glands of the body.

The colon is considered the sewage system of the body and, by abuse and neglect of proper nutrition and regularity, it can become a foul cesspool. The body then begins to become extremely acid and putrid inside. B6 is produced in the colon, Vitamin B6 being the essential ingredient to maintain digestion. There are times when we may take certain substances into our bodies which will destroy any of the Vitamin B6 we may be producing; for example — alcohol, birth control pills, coffee, radiation exposure, tobacco and narcotic drugs. Then, in order for B6 to be activated, there are other related minerals and vitamins that the body must have, such as B1 and B2, pantothenic acid and general B-complex, magnesium, potassium, linoleic acid of the fatty acid group and sodium. We may not be getting enough of these substances to produce accurate amounts of B6; however, sometimes the cause goes back to such a simple thing as stress.

The main thing we lack is the minerals, vitamins and basic good fuel to stand the stresses of life. Would you put bad gas into your new car and expect it to perform until it was finally so full of

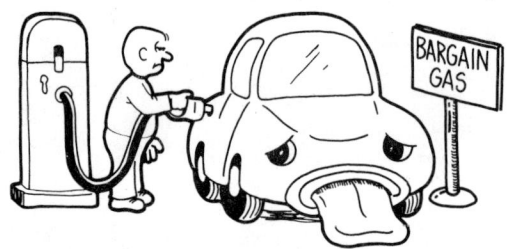

sludge it would sputter and stop? Do you expect to climb the hills of life with bad fuel? When we have had a long term stress or a traumatic experience, such as shock or grief we could not cope with, where the adrenal glands have had to produce more cortin than they were able to produce, the adrenals become exhausted to the point where they cannot produce the cortin hormone essential to the digestion of meats and starches, the same way insulin is essential to the use of sucrose sugars. At this point B6 stops its production, and lactic and uric acid begin to build. The calcium, magnesium, potassium and sodium lose their balance, causing either an excess of calcium in the blood or a deficiency in the blood, where the uric acid retains the calcium in deposit in the joints, resulting in arthritis. Other glandular diseases may also be part of the arthritis.

It has been said that death begins in the colon. A recent article in a San Francisco newspaper told the story of an elderly doctor quitting his practice at the age of 93 years. When asked for his formula for long life, his answer was, "Trust God and keep your bowels open." In our day and time the correct care of the colon has become so lost, it seems that to give even a thought to such care is quackery. It should be known by everyone that without necessary care to keep the bowels open, all kinds of degenerative diseases can result: duodenal ulcers — obstructions of the duodenum, pyloric spasms and obstruction, dilation of the stomach, gastric ulcers, cancer of the stomach and liver, atrophy of muscular wall — weakening and displacement of abdominal muscles. Colitis, appendicitis, adhesions of the intestines, enlargement of the spleen, gastritis, cancer of the pancreas, gallbladder cancer, degeneration of cirrhosis of the liver are a few diseases which are related to the digestive organs. Eventually many other parts of the body can be affected because of a toxic colon: The heart, blood vessels, nervous system, eyes, skin, muscles, joints, genital-urinary and reproductive organs, glands, etc.

ARTERIOSCLEROSIS

During the Korean war, a series of autopsies performed on soldiers with an average age of 22, revealed some degree of arteriosclerosis in three-fourths of the cases. In 12% of this group, arterial obstruction exceeded the 50% level. These men were supposed to be the "Cream of the Crop." The article states that modern warfare was tame compared to mortality rates brought about by disease: "Every year, over three times as many Americans die from cardiovascular disease as were lost in combat during the entirety of World War II and another 355,000 actually succumbed to cancer." It was stated further that, "Since 1950, per capita medical expense in the United States has more than quadrupled, yet the death rate has remained almost stationary. More medical dollars don't always result in better physical health."

THE EXOCRINE GLANDS

Another example of a modern disease, cystic fibrosis, affects all exocrine glands in varying degrees. There are three types of drugs used in treatment of cystic fibrosis:

1. oxytetracycline
2. chloramphenicol
3 erythromycin

The effects of these drugs are as follows:

1. *Chloramphenicol* — After taking this drug, serious blood dyscrasias (aplastic anemia) has been known to occur, terminating in leukemia.

2. *Erythromycin* — Dangerous taken by anyone with liver problems. May also affect the blood.

3. *Oxytetracycline* — An anti-biotic of the streptomyers type for strep infections. Any drug ending in "ine" is also narcotic and addictive.

There are three major types of cystic fibrosis affecting certain organs. The first type affects the Pancreas, Intestinal glands, Intraheptic bile ducts, Gall bladder, Sub-maxillary glands (beneath lower jaw).

The second type affects the Tracheobronchial, Brunner's glands (stomach glands — secrete intestinal juices).

The third type affects the Sweat glands, Parotid (near ear, and the muscle that closes the mouth), Salivary glands.

THE SYMPTOMS

As cystic fibrosis progresses, pulmonary lesions begin with a diffuse obstructive process, followed by infection and chronic bronchitis, with emphysema developing later. The onset of symptoms starts almost at birth, with difficult breathing and coughing, failure to gain weight, and foul-smelling stools. As the child grows, he remains extremely thin with a large protuberant abdomen. Chronic lung infections will follow with many attacks of pneumonia, and continual shortness of breath. The body seems to be so full of mucus that, in its effort to remove waste, it sweats profusely, causing a loss of large amounts of salt (sodium). In the summer, sufferers frequently develop heat prostration from the loss of sodium, which problem can sometimes be fatal.

MEDICAL TREATMENTS

In treating this disease medically, salt is added to the diet and a respiratory inhalation machine is often used, as well as such digestive medicines as pancreatic dornase, oral iodides, antibiotics to combat acute conditions, and chlortetracycline.

Masterpieces

We are all artists — in a way.
We paint pictures of our lives
  each day.
Will the colors that we use,
All rules of art abuse,
Or be blended masterfully —
  the right way?

Will the finished product hang in
  halls of fame;
Or — will we hesitate to sign
  our name?
It all depends you see,
On what we want to be.
The creation's ours,
  there's no one else to blame.

NARCOTIC ALKALOID

A narcotic alkaloid, in diseases of heavy mucus involvement, would cause the body to alkalize quickly. Continuous use of a narcotic to alkalize, allows the person to go on eating mucus-forming foods. The danger of continuous use lies in possible addiction and also in the body becoming too alkaline, to the point where the body becomes devoid of minerals — as in alkaline soil. Alkalizing the body is nature's way to heal, and to be on the alkaline side is the best way to health, provided the body is maintaining the minerals it needs. A diet heavy in concentrated foods — starches, meats and sugars — never provides enough minerals. When one drug is used to kill germs living on the refuse of such a diet (mucus), and another narcotic drug is used to alkalize, the results can be readily seen.

Cystic fibrosis is generally treated in this manner, creating not only side effects, but great dangers in taking the drugs. From my observation of natural healing methods, may I present my opinion of the cause of this disease, as well as an alternative solution, to bring about as helpful a result as possible.

PROBABLE CAUSE

The disease begins not with the child, but with the poor diet of the mother who had eaten too many mucus-forming, concentrated foods. There is also a weakness in gland function which is passed on to the child. There is a possibility of damage to the neck, causing the Choroid Plexes gland to malfunction. This is the gland which regulates the secretions of the cerebrospinal fluid.

This fluid must be maintained at a certain pressure level. When it is not correct in its functions, it has an effect on the medulla of the brain. The medulla regulates and controls the respiratory centers, the salivation, the heart, vomiting, sneezing, sweating and swallowing.

Damage to the Choroid Plexes could be the cause of the accumulation of toxic mucus waste or could be the reason this waste cannot be readily expelled from the body. Then again, the accumulation of mucus from incorrect eating could cause the Choroid Plexes to be sluggish in its regulatory function. Either way, the result is still an accumulation of mucus which is not easily removed from the body.

To be led along to the best answers, even for disease considered terminal, is an interesting and rewarding quest, if it is approached with courage and faith. The most important thing in the final analysis is not to escape death forever — no one is able to do that but rather to find the best answers possible under a given circumstance. The final score will still add up not to the winning or losing, but how well we played the game. How much pain and discomfort did we avoid and how much health did we enjoy? There is always a better way to do everything; it is just a matter of finding out what that way is. There is also a reason that we need to go through trials. The best way to seek is cheerfully, hopefully, with the faith that you will find the answers.

*LADY SLIPPER

The herb which acts on the medulla and the choroid plexes is Lady Slipper *(Cypripeduim pubescens)*. This wonderful herb is one of the most expensive botanicals on the market. It is a relaxant herb, antispasmodic, nervine and tonic, but acts primarily on the medulla, helping to regulate breathing, sweating, saliva and heart functions. It is also called "moccasin flower." The plant grows in moist woodlands in many parts of Europe, Asia, and America. The blossoms have a sac-like lip shaped like a moccasin or slipper.

Lady Slipper, along with other cleansing herbs such as burdock, poke root, licorice, and mandrake, in a formula, and with a mild food diet of fruits, vegetables and lots of Vitamin C, will allow the waste to be easily moved out of the body. It would logically follow that when a person has such weaknesses, it would be essential to live on a good diet continually in order to maintain general health and often use the cleansing, maintaining herbs. This approach is a much more sensible way to maintain life with *cystic fibrosis* than to take dangerous drugs.

Whether or Not

Whether we do
   or
Whether we don't
Can make a big difference in life.
Whether we will
   or
Whether we won't
Will determine what error is rife.

Drugs

CONSIDERATION of the terrible deformities caused by mothers taking wonder drugs shows the results of a serious, often deadly, mistaken trust in the use of drugs. We are urged to have our children innoculated, vaccinated, and given oral vaccines. However, thinking people who have observed the devastating effect of drugs upon our society are looking for alternative solutions and finding effective help without side effects through the use of herbs.

We are living in a time when over the past fifty years some people have been literally drugged to death. Many have become so upset by this fast-moving society that they feel the need for something to quiet their nerves. Medically stated side effects prove that certain drugs taken over a period of time will induce mental imbalance. Drugs tend to suppress the efforts of nature to heal, by treating the effect and ignoring the cause.

Using the generic or chemical names, we shall take a look at some of the major suppressant drugs, the downers, the nerve relaxants and sedatives, and see what they do to the body.

Many of these drugs mentioned are used in compounds (commercial brands) in conjunction with other dangerous ingredients, such as caffeine, codeine, and aspirin.

Barbituric acid is one of these dangerous drugs. Chemists make it by heating a substance related to malonic acid and urea (a compound found in urine, blood and lymph of man and other mammals). U.S. physicians use more than 25 kinds of barbituates in medical practice.

Belladonna

There are approximately 21 commercial brands of belladonna on the market. Belladonna is the deadly night shade plant; people have died from eating the berries.

The alkaloid derived from this plant is called *Scopolamie*, which the eye doctor uses as drops to relax eye muscles and causes pupils to dilate. It is also taken internally as a relaxant.

Dangers: When used where there is hypothyroidism, myxedema, glaucoma, prostatic hypertrophy, or increased size of prostate gland, and bladder and liver obstruction can develop. This drug can cause blindness, death, and hallucinations.

Caffeine is a *cranial vasoconstrictor* often used for migraine headache. This drug is known to be dangerous where there are heart trouble, liver or kidney problems, hypertension, or pregnancy. People still continue to drink coffee, one source of caffeine, on a daily basis, along with food and treat coffee as if it were a wholesome food. Caffeine is also added to other dangerous drugs and is often used for a headache. Hypertension is often the cause of headache, and even the medical books say caffeine should not be used in cases of hypertension.

Chloral Hydrate

Rx names: *Noctec, Beta-Chlor-Somas.*

This drug is caustic and is a poison which can eventually paralyze the central nervous system. If chloral hydrate is mixed with alcohol is called knock out drops or a "Mickey Finn," since it causes immediate sleep. It creates a reaction similar to strong alcohol intoxication when used alone: drowsiness, slurred speech, confusion, uncoordination, and respiratory depression.

Dangers: When used where there is cardiac disease, kidney or liver disease it is addictive. This drug is made up of carbon, chlorine, hydrogen and oxygen. In this particular combination it is a caustic poison. Chloral hydrate is used today, obtained from illicit sources, by some young people, and is a very dangerous drug.

Morphine

Rx name: *morphine sulfate*, U.S.P. It is used for pain and has a poison in the alkaloid form. Morphine is derived from the Opium poppy, the same source as Heroin. Morphine is found in many cough syrups. This drug causes lethargy, drowsiness, confusion euphoria or an abnormal false feeling of buoyant vigor and well-being, along with slurred speech, flushing skin on face, neck and chest, vomiting, and constricted pupils. Morphine causes chronic constipation, is addictive, and also causes a forcible, rapid pulse which then becomes slow and feeble.

Respiratory depression becomes shallow and the body skin, pale, cold, and moist. The person becomes difficult to arouse.

Scars or abesses develop at injection sites (called "needle marks") after continued use.

Dangers: In thyroid disease, respiratory problems can develop, as well as kidney and liver problems, since morphine is a poison. An overdose will cause death by slowing the lungs until they stop functioning.

Morphine addicts make up the largest group of drug addicts in the United States. Horace Sutton said that death due to narcotics has risen five fold in New York, from 200 in 1960 to more than a thousand in 1969. The Board of Education estimates that there were 22,000 Heroin users in New York City's secondary schools (as of 1970). Approximately 150,000 Americans were on the drug at that time. The percentage of users is increasing fast and Horace Sutton also said we had only 10 years from 1970 to doomsday because of drug use in America. We have already used nine of those 10 years.

Pentobarbital

Pentobarbitol is another barbituate that depresses the nervous system. It is used with sodium as a short-acting sedative. This drug causes a similar intoxication to that produced by alcohol, bringing drowsiness, confusion, uncoordination, depressed pulse rate and low blood pressure, mildly dilated pupils, and respiratory depression.

Dangers: Used in the presence of liver problems, kidney weakness, and glaucoma, it becomes extremely dangerous.

The *side effects* are blurred vision, dry mouth, lethargy, circulatory collapse, and respiratory depression. Pentobarbitol is often used as a suppository and can become habit-forming in any use.

Phenobarbital (or phenylethyobarbital acid).

This well-known drug, with some 52 name brands on the market, has a depressive effect on motor nerve areas. It is often used for spasms of a gastrointestinal nature associated with spastic colitis or spastic colon constipation, epilepsy, and nervous disorders.

It should not be used for glaucoma, liver disease, kidney, bladder obstructions for elderly or weak persons, unstable cardiovascular status, ulcerated colitis, myasthenia-gravis, diabetes, hypothyroidism.

Dangers: Since phenobarbital decreases sweating, there is danger in its use in a warm environment.

It can cause blurred vision, increased ocular tension, pain, mental confusion, renal kidney retention, heart palpatations, dry mouth and throat, and when used regularly it becomes habit forming and can cause impotence and suppressed lactation.

Phenol is the other part of this drug, a coal tar product dangerous because of its rapid corrosive action on body tissues. Phenol is poison if taken internally, and even a five percent solution used on the skin can cause local gangrene. These two chemicals together make phenobarbital.

Secobarbital

Secobarbital is often called by users on the illicit market, "goof balls," "barbs," and "downers."

Seconal, its prescription name, is a habit-forming barbiturate which is often used as a sedative for pain of arthritis and neuritis, often used on wounds.

This drug acts on the senses the same way as other barbiturates.

Dangers: When used where there is glaucoma, liver, or kidney disease, peptic ulcers, or a low convulsive threshold, secobarbital can be dangerous.

When the drugs mentioned here are studied carefully, remembering that only the generic chemical names have been used and not the many prescriptive names of commercial brands, one can easily see that in order to take pain killers and relaxant sedative drugs it is essential to have a good heart, a sound liver and kidneys, and be in top physical condition.

All poisons are supposed to detoxify in the liver and be carried out of the body, but any time a poison is taken into the body, the heart is weakened. Therefore, one can now see the difference between an herb relaxant and a drug. To take herbs is to add good food and the nutritional value of their vitamins and minerals to

Survival

Every creature on the earth
will fight to stay alive.
Let's be sure that what we fight for,
makes us worthy to survive.

the body, thereby increasing the vital force rather than depressing the energy and ability to throw off the body's wastes. Drugs also leave a residue of toxic waste poison which weakens rather than builds. This residue is what eventually causes side effects.

Think about exactly how suppressing drugs work on the nervous system. Consider the importance of the nervous system. Without a nervous system man would be a senseless, motionless, thoughtless nothing. Because of the nervous system he senses, knows, remembers, conveys, communicates, moves, breathes, finds meaning in the printed page, and regulates hundreds of automatic activities. Nothing can approach the complexity of the human brain and nervous system. With all of man's ingenuity to build computers, he cannot come near the marvels of the human communication system.

When the nervous system is even vaguely understood in all its far-reaching infinite aspects, how can man disbelieve in God? There has to be a greater intelligence creating such infinite beauty and wonder as the human body, where messages are carried as invisibly as conversation on a telephone wire.

From the cry of a hungry baby, to the prick of a pin, every stimulus causes a message to be sent to the brain. The stimuli neurons are always busy transmitting nerve impulses from one part of our structure to another with split second accuracy, unless we do something to interfere by overreacting, closing off, suppressing, or stopping the chain reaction. When we accumulate a buildup of toxic waste, causing interference or allowing negative thoughts to pinch off the nerve wire (the way the arteries can be closed down by stress and upset, as in high blood pressure), we shut off our ability to preserve, know, learn, feel, and live.

The scare tactics used to get people to take drugs are again being used to keep people from using herbs, but those who use herbs and find the marvelous, inexpensive help that comes from the use of God's medicines are not impressed by the latest propaganda against them. Herbs have been tried and tested since time began and used with helpful results through all ages with only the exception of the past fifty years. During this period the knowledge of herbs has been suppressed. There has gone with this suppression a hope that there was such a thing as a cure-all drug that man could invent for each disease. Unfortunately, often drug using people were playing guinea pig for the drug industry and were not kept informed as to the potential hazards.

Even the lowly aspirin, according to the medical books, "accounts for about half of the drug deaths in children." If we are among those who reason and think for ourselves, we must conclude that there is an easier, better way to heal an already sick body than with destructive drugs.

Herbs

HERBS are the logical answer because they do not cause slurred speech, intoxication, pain, poisoning, blurred vision, uncoordination, respiratory depression, hallucinations, or psychosis. They do not injure the heart, liver, or kidneys. They are pure foods: Mild herbs are God's medicines. Isn't it time we learned about them again?

Herbs are not new to the world. Anyone supposing that herbs are unscientific, has not studied the history of medicine. There is, in this country, an awakening of our herbal cultural heritage which can save future generations if it is not stifled by the ignorance of the average lay person who often allows others to decide the fate of his or her own body, no matter what. This seemingly new awakening is but part of an old heritage which has been suppressed for the past fifty years. This awakening is growing in strength as people find that they are tired of being sick and are tired of paying the high cost of being sick. People are reaching out to preventive medicine and to herbal medicine and are finding their answers in two small words, *"it works."*

Herbs are not as pleasant a replacement for nutrients as those found in fruits and vegetables, grains, and seeds and were not intended to replace more palatable food. Their function is to regulate organs and glands, correct the balance, and cleanse the cells. Over a century ago Americans started the most costly experiment in history — living on refined foods — and at the same time discontinuing the general use of herbs, using synthetic drugs for medicine instead. This has proven to be a disaster to the general health of the nation.

When we consider the wonders that occur with herbal use, as well as the over-all nutritious value of each herb, without the dangerous side-effects of drugs, we begin to marvel at the simplicity of God's medicines. Each herb can be taken alone specifically, or used with others, each herb lending its own strength and power to soothe and heal sicknesses of the human body.

One day we will know every intricate part of each of these wondrous herbs and why each part is relative to the other. In the meantime we accept the fact that they do work; we give gratitude to a great and wise God who provided simple, workable methods to relieve suffering. The reward of proof lies in the fact that herbs do work — and without any side-effect.

We are fast approaching the time when herbs will be recognized for their great value to the life of the diabetic and the person who suffers kidney failure. We are quickly reaching an important turning point in medicine, when men of science are reaching out to old time-worn methods and finding it is more helpful to suffering humanity to abandon many of the ideological traditions accepted over the past fifty years and return to nature's own medicines.

The apostle Paul, in his effort to unite the Roman church, wrote: "Him that is weak in the faith receive ye, but not to doubtful disputations." (Romans 14:1) He then says in the following verse: "For one believeth that he may eat all things; another who is weak, eateth herbs —"

Some people believe this scripture connects weakness in the faith with the use of herbs. I believe that there is a great difference between being weak physically and being weak in the faith. Could we, if we had enough faith, live on cake, candy and ice cream day and night? Could we, if we had enough faith, drink all the liquor and smoke all the cigarettes we wanted with impunity? Can we blindly go along on so-called faith, eating all the sugar and foodless foods we want, disregarding the laws of good health? When there are laws which operate in mathematics, science, physiology, spirituality, and sociology, could it be possible that there is no law concerning what we eat?

I know a man whose doctor told him he could eat all the sugar he wanted, which he does boastfully because the doctor said it was okay. It has not occurred to him or his doctor that the fifteen years or more of a chronic skin disease could be in any way related to his heavy consumption of sugar.

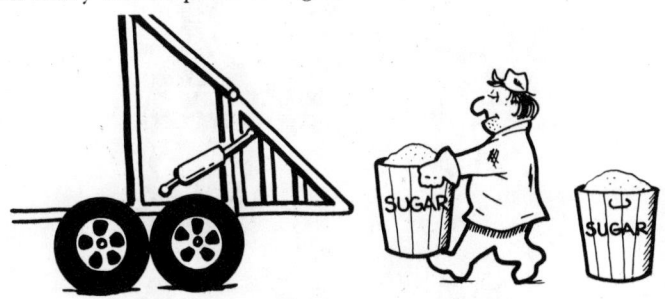

If a chemist combined certain materials in his test tube, he could blow himself into outer space. Is there no rule for the human test tube? Can we, by faith, eat anything?

As I study the wonder and order in the herb kingdom and the exact, perfectly consistent reaction each herb has in human bodies of all sizes, I know that Paul was saying all those whose *bodies* were weak eat herbs.

Our medicine should be able to add to our vital force rather than depressing and reducing the body's energy ability to throw off waste and disease.

Much of the chronic disease we know today has been the result of such suppression by reducing the body's ability to throw off waste, often causing the sufferer to become permanently ill.

Every naturopathic or natural healing doctor has known that all acute disease is the body's attempt to eliminate pathological disease-causing filth from itself. They have also known that chronic disease is filth waste, mucus lodged somewhere in the body unable to eliminate because of continual wrong diet or negative thought patterns, tensions, and organic malfunctions. Non-poisonous herbs are considered *food* as well as medicine. They do not suppress or interfere with the body's effort to cleanse and heal itself, but rather assist by adding vitality and soothing, cleansing abilities by never producing any harmful side effects.

Many young people are not looking to science to change the world situation. These youth are really leading us in the direction of natural healing and natural foods. For this we can be grateful especially when such changes have been painful and traumatic experiences for so many youngsters involved in illicit drug use. No changes are ever made without struggle and pain. It seems to take the young and inexperienced to venture into the unknown and take the bumps.

Among the adults are those die-hards who cling to the old hope that medical science will discover a new drug which will allow man

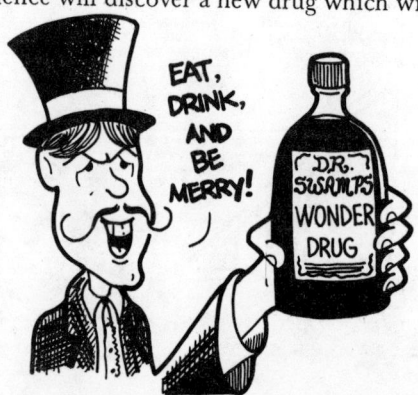

to "eat, drink, and be merry" while still maintaining good health. This has been a myth for years. Along with the young drug culture of the past decade, many intelligent people are deciding that the only road to real health is to live by the laws upon which good health is predicated.

People everywhere are becoming disenchanted with drugs and the high cost of dying and are looking for alternative solutions. And they are finding them in the wonderful herbs growing all over the world. People are re-discovering that food and herbs are the medicines God intended man to use to maintain optimal health.

It is becoming fashionable to dine at the new organic restaurants springing up all over the country on sprouts and Bible bread sandwiches. There are even Bible bread stands, like hamburger stands, arousing young people's interest. The center of a Bible bread sandwich is a mock meat made of garbanzos and sesame. The Bible bread, or pocket bread, is also filled with herbs, lettuce, and tomatoes.

Celebrities, movie stars, and many well-known people have joined the health kick and are discovering that it works. Good health is becoming a marvelous experience. Athletes are turning to natural foods, vitamins, and bee pollen for strength and energy, rejecting high protein diets. Doctors at medical conventions are finally concluding that what we eat has something to do with our health.

Even in a sagging economy, herb companies have grown phenomenally — comparable to the growth made by the drug companies of the 30's and 40's. The return to herbal medicine is the "in" thing. Realizing the destructive power of drugs those who formerly embraced drugs are now embracing nature's way and experiencing the same dramatic changes — only this time, for the better. Just as they pursued revolutionary concepts then, they are realizing, today, a revolution in their own health and well-being is, perhaps, part of the answer to curing the world's ills.

Reflecting on my 30 years involvement in the natural way of living, I remember it was always with reservation that I dared to tell anyone about my way of life. People used to look both ways before going into a health food store for fear a friend might see them. The label "health nut" was coined out of this minority difference.

The general concensus that chemical drugs cure was so ingrained, that I dared not rock anyone's boat in those days by suggesting that there was an easier, better, less expensive way to health. It is difficult for me to understand why some people hang on so bulldoggedly to medicine when documented "natural" successes are so prevalent.

For many years, studies have indicated how to feed and keep our dogs, cats, and horses healthy. Now it is time for us to learn how to feed and keep humans healthy. Many people are aware of this need and anyone who is not in step with the times may get lost in the shuffle if medical treatment steps aside for preventive medicine to take its place.

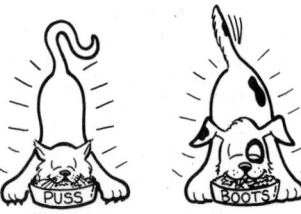

There is a group of people at the present who are claiming that herbs have no "good" value, so that herbs can be classed as drugs and kept under strict medical control. Research has been done on many herbs and their values are well-known. There is much yet to do in order to maintain herbs in the classification of food (which they in fact are) and still allow us to choose which herbs and foods we will use in our diets. When we consider the degeneration of our civilization, much of which has been the direct result of drugs, it becomes time to re-evaluate past misinformation and begin a quest for health. wisdom, and a better way. To say there is no food value in herbs would be to say that animals could not exist on the grasses and herbs of the fields. When most of the vitamin research has been done only on animals, it would be absurd to try to explain herbs away as having no food value.

Herbs, along with good fruits and vegetables, could become the healers of a sick society, if people would but seek these answers with open minds and prayerful hearts.

Whether we take herbs or drugs to calm the nerves, we must first look to our mental attitudes if we are ever to find complete answers. We must consider health in both mind and body if results are to be permanent.

There must be something wrong with people who want only to treat the effects of a disease but have no desire to find the cause. This creates the visual picture of a tap running in the kitchen sink with a clogged drain, causing water to spill all over the floor. Rather than shut off the tap and open the drain, scientific intellectuals stand around with a mop and mop up the water until the flood becomes a catastrophe. Then, when they give up in despair, they give us the time-worn phrase: "There is nothing more we can do."

When we watch the miracles that happen because of using certain herbs, could it be that such herbs are merely supplying much needed vitamins and minerals in a concentrated form? Could it be also, that they clean out the sludge and give better performance to our engines? We know that herbs do something remarkable and with no side effects, but there has not been enough research about the vitamin value of herbs. May I challenge researchers to seek out these things? In the meantime, here is some information gathered about vitamin values in herbs.

Vitamin A

Vitamin A has a strengthening effect on the arteries, combats infection, increases vitality, aids in body growth with bones and teeth, and also assists the body in the use of iodine.

SOURCES: Cayenne, Dandelion, Eyebright, Grape leaves, Lambs quarter, Okra pods, Paprika, Parsley, Red raspberry, Violet.

Alcohol, Coffee, Cortisone, excessive unnatural iron and mineral oil destroy Vitamin A, and a Vitamin D deficiency inhibits the correct use of Vitamin A.

Vitamin B1

B1 changes glucose into energy or fat and is known as the memory, starch-sugar metabolism vitamin and aids in resistance to noise and pain.

B1 is destroyed by alcohol, coffee, sugar, tobacco, narcotic drugs.

SOURCES: Bladderwrack, Dandelion, Dulse, Fenugreek, Grape leaves, Kelp, Okra, Red raspberry.

Vitamin B2

B2 brings oxygen to the eyes; milk sugar (lactose) increases the need for B2 unless fat is adequate in diet.

SOURCES: Bladderwrack, Dulse, Fenugreek, Kelp, Saffron, Wild Rose hips. B2 is also destroyed by alcohol, sugar, coffee, narcotic drugs and tobacco.

Vitamin B6

B6 is essential in using fatty acids, linoleic acids and amino acids from protein. It also assists in hormonal metabolism in the thyroid gland. Vitamin B6 is made in the colon (when the colon is sick, yogurt and acidophilus culture are helpful to its production). It is destroyed by alcohol, birth control pills, coffee, radiation exposure, tobacco, narcotic drugs and constipation.

Vitamin B6 Deficiencies

It may be interesting to the reader to know some of the symptoms of the lack of vitamin B6:

Certain eczema in babies	Bed wetting
Acne	Bladder retention
Psoriasis	Tooth decay
Dermatitis wrinkles	Sinus problems
Fainting easily	Water retention
Sore mouth	Toxemia in pregnancy
Muscle cramps	Vomiting after surgery
Neuritis	Hypoglycemia
Hair loss	Nervous disorders
Facial oiliness	

Vitamin B12

Vitamin B12 is for the glands. Folic acid is needed to use B12 (phenobarbital, dilantin and heat destroy folic acid). This is a good reason for using fresh raw cold-pressed oils, fruits and nuts. Essential in the assimilation of meat protein and in gland restoration.

SOURCES: Alfalfa, Bladderwrack, Dulse, Kelp.

Destroyed by too many laxatives, alcohol, coffee, tobacco and narcotic drugs.

Vitamin C

Vitamin C is known as the anti-poison and anti-inflammation vitamin, useful in all acute diseases.

SOURCES: Elder berries, Rose hips, Watercress.

Tobacco, antibiotics, aspirin and cortisone destroy Vitamin C.

Vitamin D

Essential to the use of calcium by the body.
SOURCES: Alfalfa, Lettuce, Sunshine or sunlight.
Mineral oil destroys Vitamin D.

Vitamin E

Among other things, Vitamin E is an anti-sterility vitamin and it is essential to growth. This is why red raspberry is so useful during pregnancy. It is essential for the assimilation of Vitamins A, C, D and K by the body.

SOURCES: Red raspberry, Rose hips.

Like Vitamin D, it is destroyed by mineral oil and birth control pills.

MINERALS

Following are some of the major minerals.

Calcium

Calcium is necessary for the formation of sound teeth and bones, lactation and pregnancy, oxygen to the brain, nerve impulse transmission, muscle contraction and promotes clotting.

SOURCES: Alfalfa (34.9 percent), Chamomile, Dandelion, Nettle, Plantain, Red raspberry.

Alcohol, cortisone, salt, sugar and coffee destroy calcium.

Iodine

SOURCES: Black walnut, Bladderwrack, Dulse, Kelp.

Iron

There are many natural sources of iron. Synthetic iron is an aluminum derivative that is very harmful to the human body.

SOURCES: Alfalfa (1.30 percent, very high for a trace mineral), Burdock (High in iron), Dandelion, Red raspberry, Yellow dock.

Magnesium

SOURCES: Dandelion (good source, has the same effect as chemical alkalizers from a magnesium salt source, without leaving the residue.) Leaf lettuce, Mullein, Parsley, Watercress.

Phosphorus

SOURCES: Alfalfa, Chickweed, Licorice, Red raspberry, Watercress.

Potassium

Essential to strong muscle tone. Potassium regulates the fluids of the body and works in cooperation with the Thyroid Gland. When there is a correct potassium balance, the body will not retain fluid unless there is damage to the kidneys.

SOURCES: Dandelion, Harrow, Mistletoe, Parsley, Plantain, Watercress.

The vitamin and mineral value of food or herbs cannot be the same as an amount measured and laboratory tested because one food or herb may have been grown in better soil than another, making the potency higher. We can, however, know which foods or herbs are highest in known values.

HERBS FOR PARASITES

Parasites belong either to the plant or animal kingdom.

In his book *Medical Parasitology,* Dr. William G. Swaitz, M.D., defines parasitism as, "The association of two specifically different organisms in which one partner lives on or within the other and feeds at its expense."

Parasites vary in their effect on their host. Sometimes they seem to be harmless. The parasites considered dangerous are called "pathogens." The parasite which causes malarial fevers is an example of this. Many protozoans (one celled animals) are parasites, such as a certain type of amoeba which can destroy the lining of the intestines of humans, producing a painful and serious disease called "amoebic dysentery." If this disease continues unchecked, the body can become dehydrated and eventually the bowel will bleed and ulcerate.

Animals are subject to such protozoans, which can invade the blood of mammals and cause diseases such as malaria, lupus, and Texas cattle fever. Blood-sucking insects and ticks can pick up parasites which have infected one animal, and then transport them on to another animal or human.

Some parasites, such as flatworms and roundworms, can cause serious damage and can often kill their hosts. There is one type of flatworm called a "fluke" which lives and grows quite large in the intestines, liver, lungs or blood of animals and man.

The tapeworm is another parasite which matures in the intestines, attaching itself to the intestinal wall with what appears to be suckers or hooks. The tapeworm absorbs digested foods from its host, but the hookworm is the most harmful since it lives in the intestines and it feeds on the blood of the host.

There are many forms of external skin parasites, such as ticks and mites. The skin is irritated by such bites, but the spread of disease is far more serious than the bite. Ticks are blamed for having spread Rocky Mountain spotted fever, yellow fever, African sleeping sickness and typhus fever.

It has been recently discovered that cancer may also be caused by a parasite. This parasite was identified by Dr. Virginia Livingston, M.D., and was written about in her book, *Cancer, A New Breakthrough*. She calls the parasite the **progeniter cryptocide**. This parasite begins as the lepra or tubercular bacillus and changes form to become the cancer parasite.

Bacteria

Bacteria are one-celled organisms. Most kinds of bacteria must live off the refuse of man's or animal's bodies. There are three main types of bacteria:

Bacilli are rod-shaped, often grow in long chains.
Cocci are spherical and grow in grape-like clusters.
Spirilla are spirally curved.

One bacterium can produce over 16,000,000 new bacteria in twenty-four hours. The bacteria which cause disease live and grow like parasites in the soft tissue, blood and bones, or in the stems and fruits of plants. Bacteria are involved in contagious diseases such as scarlet fever, whooping cough, tetanus, diphtheria, pneumonia, gonorrhea, tuberculosis, typhoid fever, syphilis, leprosy, meningitis, plague, measles, mumps, chicken pox, etc. These are generally called acute diseases because they are associated with acute pain and fever; however, some are chronic or long term.

Salmonella

Salmonella is a microscopic organism which can spread throughout the body, reaching such high counts that the afflicted person becomes acutely sick with what is commonly called cholera. Many people today have the intermittent fever of cholera, but are given antibiotics and never told what their problem has been.

Trichinosis

This disease is brought about by eating infected, undercooked pork. The trichina is a tiny worm that infects pigs. The larvae, after burrowing into the intestinal wall of the pig, then enters its blood vessels. The blood carries the larvae on to the muscles where these tiny worms spread into the muscle fiber and live. Then, if the pig is eaten by man, the cycle begins again in the human.

Often people have trichinosis and do not even realize that the symptoms they feel are caused by these internal worms. It is often difficult for a physician to diagnose trichinosis because the symptoms, such as headache, fever, sore muscles, and swollen eyes, and painful breathing, are so similar to other diseases.

Science tells us that the parasite or the germ is the cause of disease, but it is my opinion that the exact opposite is true. The parasite comes as the result of too much of the kind of food which it can feed on — both in plants and animals.

If the body is well-nourished and clean inside, parasites and germs cannot multiply and grow. We do not have maggots on our sink when we keep it clean and neither will we have worms in our bodies if we keep them clean.

Often when people try to live on a cleaner, or cleansing diet, they cannot stay on it because the parasites within are crying for the kind of junk foods upon which they live and grow. Usually the body must be cleansed of parasites separately, while the cleansing is in process. Because the parasites hang on to the mucus in which they live, the body cannot be made well even in a fasting or semi-fasting situation. The parasites must first be killed; then the mucus in which they were living will pour forth out of the body, much like a healing crisis.

To kill the parasites in the body is not enough, however. A total change in diet is essential if a person expects to maintain health and remain free of such infestation. The body must be maintained on healthful (organically grown, if possible) foods to insure needed vitamins and minerals. Devitalized junk foods, which deteriorate into mucus (fine food for the parasite), should not be eaten.

As we watch the bacterial changes in nature, it should occur to us that the only way not to become a part of decay is to live the rules of good nutrition. We know that by using the right herbs we can safely kill and remove parasites from the body. The big challenge, however, is to maintain such a clean body that there is no food for parasites.

Some other herbs which kill parasites or expel worms from the body are:

Aspen	Pink Root
Bearsfoot	Pumpkin Seed
Black Walnut	Senna
Blue Flag	Sorrel
Dulse	Tansy
Kelp	Wintergreen
Mandrake	Wood Sage

There are several types of parasites, including malaria and lupus, which can be killed with Black Walnut — approximately four to six capsules a day. Chapparal is another herb which kills parasites — approximately four to nine capsules a day. People used to de-worm their children; now they only de-worm their dogs. Often the dog dies from the harsh de-worming drugs. Maybe that is why children are not de-wormed any more.

Garlic is one of the best herbs for pin worms, and it can be used in a garlic enema. Garlic can also be taken in pearls. Natural herbs and garlic are not dangerous, but helpful in ridding the body of parasites and germs. When a child has any contagious disease a garlic emena will help to kill not only parasites in the bowel, but will kill germs throughout the body and shorten the duration of the disease. When using herbs for children, one should always use half of a regular adult dose — up to about 12 years old.

Unless we keep our bodies clean by maintaining good nutrition, we are making ourselves into perfect feeding grounds for parasites. Herbs are the perfect and natural way to first cleanse ourselves of the parasites that live on us, so that we can then live beautifully.

ALFALFA FOR EVERYONE

We were a poor family (mother, father, and five children), and like so many others during the Depression, we enjoyed few luxuries. However, we did have a rich heritage of wonderful truths, as is said in the modern vernacular, "laid upon us." One was alfalfa mint tea. I reflect with great love and respect upon the times when I was sick and Dad was my doctor. He did not believe in orthodox doctors, but in faith healings and the use of natural methods. I can see him as he began to doctor mé, hurriedly rushing in the door, arms laden with sacks of oranges, grapefruits, and lemons. Then he would stand for more than an hour at the sink, squeezing them all into juice, while giving my mother instructions to have me drink only juice all day — with the exception of alfalfa mint tea and honey.

The pungent aroma of alfalfa mint tea always revives nostalgic childhood memories of hot steaming tea with honey. Dad would always say, as he handed us a glass of alfalfa mint tea, "Alfalfa is the best alkaline food you can eat, and has more minerals and vitamins than anything else. It grows deep into the ground and picks up all the good possible, so drink it all down."

Alfalfa is rich in Vitamins A, C, D, B2, B6, E and K. Tests have shown it to contain remarkable amounts of minerals: calcium (34.9%), iron (1.30%), phophorus, potassium, magnesium, chlorine, sodium and silicon. All these are relative to the use of calcium in the body. Alfalfa may be the most natural aid to calcium assimilation, containing all components naturally related to minerals which cause calcium to be utilized by the body. It has a way of correcting hypercalcemia and osteoporosis problems caused by an imbalance in the glands. Alfalfa contains eight essential enzymes: the fat splitting enzyme, lipase; the enzyme which acts upon starches, amylase; the blood clotting enzyme, coagulase; and protase, which helps to digest protein , among others. The author feels that alfalfa has a definite effect on growth, not only because of the mineral and vitamin supply, but because it is a pituitary hormone, acting on the pituitary gland. The pituitary gland regulates growth. If the gland malfunctions during growth periods, a dwarf or a giant may result. Children who do not seem to grow or thrive could be lacking this essential hormone.

Arthritis

The great value of alfalfa with regard to arthritis is known, but is not clearly defined. It seems to work like celery juice in drawing calcium from the joints back into circulation and in relieving the pain. Alfalfa grows easily in many soil conditions as well as in varying climates. It is one of the richest feed crops for livestock, especially for dairy cows. Man can soon discover, to his amazement, alfalfa's great value as a human food and medicine.

It will be interesting to watch for further testing from those men who have ventured out of the field of medicinal drugs into the herb kingdom to find answers to arthritis, since the most common treatment today for arthritis is aspirin. When we recognize the deadly effects of aspirin on the body, it is refreshing to note the scientific studies done by these medical doctors from an herbal approach. There has been increasing scientific research into alfalfa, and soon we will more fully understand alfalfa's curative properties.

Through the years I have learned to be even more grateful for this wonderful, nourishing, medicinal herb, alfalfa. Raising my children, I learned that alfalfa mint tea would stop colic, and with no other help, would clear up a cold in a short time. This grand herb did exactly as Dad had taught me; it alkalized the body. It also helped my body make the best milk for my nursing babies.

A few years ago I became especially grateful for alfalfa when I learned that it is a pituitary hormone. My oldest married daughter learned she was afflicted with terminal Cushing's disease. (Lack of pituitary hormone.) Having learned about hormone herbs, I tried to find the proper herbal cure. I studied all I could find about the pituitary gland, and finally determined that no one, not even the old herbalists, could give me the answer. I realized that prayer was the only answer. I cried and prayed for some time. One day the answer came loud and clear – alfalfa! This seemed to be too simple, so I continued to pray. It seems that sometimes we pray, but aren't still long enough to hear the answer. One day, while I was quietly meditating in a warm tub of water, the answer came. This time I was able to put together all the things I had studied. ACTH is the drug used for Cushing's disease which has a protein molecule. At last I realized that alfalfa has a protein molecule as well! The whole thing came into clear focus in my mind, and I knew that alfalfa was the answer I sought. My daughter took alfalfa pills for three months, and when she had her next check-up, her hormone was in balance. She was also taking other related hormone herbs, but alfalfa was the herb which brought the disease to subjugation. The doctor told her, "Whatever you are taking, you'd better continue with it."

There have been many articles written about alfalfa sprouts, which are at the top of the list of nutritious foods: live, raw and unspoiled by chemical fertilizers and sprays. Much of today's lettuce and salad crops are badly sprayed. People who try to live on a vegetarian diet, in which they eat large amounts of lettuce and salad vegetables, may become poisoned. Alfalfa sprouts are a fine addition to a sandwich or a salad, and are also very tasty eaten alone.

Hormones

These sprouts, however, do not supply the hormone contained in the whole herb plant. It has been my experience that alfalfa is a hormone herb which affects the parathyroid glands, along with natural iodine. Whenever one has a twitchy muscle, it is usually due to a lack of magnesium, but it may also be the parathyroid glands. There are four of these tiny glands, situated like small beads superficially embedded on the back side of the thyroid gland. The hormones secreted are parathormone and calcitonin, which function to maintain a stable concentration of calcium in the blood. Whenever blood calcium levels are too low, parathormone activates the transfer of calcium from bone to blood until the calcium level is returned to normal. Calcitonin is released when there is an excess of calcium in the blood. The most prominent symptom is an excessive neuromuscular excitability manifesting itself in twiching wrists and foot spasms.

Muscle spasms over the entire body, which cause convulsions, are often mistaken for epilepsy. There is both a hyper and a hypo type of parathyroid difficulty, and alfalfa and iodine work equally well on both. Hyper is the thin type and hypo is the fat type. Hyper requires a small dose; hypo requires a larger dose, small amounts being four to six iodine kelp tablets or six to 10 alfalfa tablets; larger doses being from 10 to 40 kelp tablets and from 10 to 20 alfalfa tablets. With Cushing's disease, 20 to 40 or more alfalfa tablets are needed to control it.

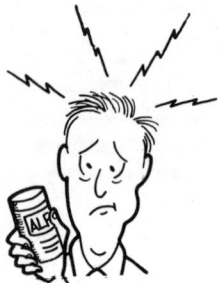

Occasionally, we find a person whose pituitary gland is so activated by the use of alfalfa that it causes him an immediate headache, the way black cohosh does when the body does not need it. This headache leaves almost as quickly as it comes and is caused by too much activation of the gland, which creates a swelling of the tiny pituitary gland that has no room in the head to expand. This is only a momentary experience, but it is a good gauge of whether or not that much alfalfa is needed. When one begins to use herbs, he soon discovers that there is no need to fear such little experiences, for there are no real side effects among the mild herbs. Of course, the use of deadly or narcotic herbs is not condoned.

There are many kinds of alfalfa, and plant breeders have developed other varieties which are suitable for growing in certain climates. Varieties that are winter-hardy and will resist aphid and bacterial wilt disease are being developed. If a strict standard of organic gardening were established in the production of alfalfa, no insecticides would be necessary. Alfalfa grows 12 to 40 inches in height and can grow from two to 25 feet into the ground in search of water. It also may be grown in a fairly dry climate as an ideal crop.

Farmers have learned that alfalfa enriches the soil, restoring nitrogen to soil depleted by growing corn and wheat. Alfalfa returns to the soil elements used up by other crops. Alfalfa is a perennial plant, which seems to die with the approach of winter. When the warm weather arrives, however, new green shoots appear and will reappear for the next three to six years. It is a hardy, valuable herb, important to the American economy as well as to the economies of Central and South America, Asia, Africa, Australia, and Europe. In Europe, it is called lucerne. Farmers have learned that alfalfa has great nutritional value, and that cows fed on alfalfa give larger quantities of very rich milk. There are few, if any, plants which can compete with alfalfa as a soil builder. When the crop is turned under, besides adding organic nutrients to the soil, dead tops and roots of the plant loosen and aerate the soil, helping it to hold water.

BLACK COHOSH FOR THE WOMAN

During the past few years, with more female surgery and more women taking the pill, the use of estrogen has become quite common as an aid to physical and emotional balance for these women. Those who have sought escape from emotional problems because of a lack of the necessary amount of estrogen being produced in their bodies have discovered to their dismay, that the side effects of the drug are almost worse than doing without the drug. We read of reports of more uterine cancer because of the use of estrogen. This is a rather frightening prospect for a woman who has no apparent choice other than to have her female organs removed. She has nothing to look forward to but increased nervousness, emotional instability, and possible eventual cancer. Would we be compromising or would we be wise if we began to look for alternative solutions to this dilemma? If there were an herb which would allow the woman who has had all of her female organs removed, the probable option of maintaining herself without side effect, this solution would be highly desirable even though she had to take the herb for the rest of her life.

When our grandmothers were young, there was a woman named Lydia Pinkham who advertised a patented herbal formula with the slogans, *"A baby in every bottle"* or *"For Female complaint."* Still located in her old building, there are files with thousands of unsolicited letters thanking her for her wonderful formula. It was not by accident that her formula helped woman. Of the four herbs in the formula, one was one-half estrogen. Following the discovery of estrogen, a group of scientists verified this statement when they decided to see if Lydia Pinkham had anything of value.

Black Cohosh is a hormone type herb which has numerous uses. One of the botanical names for black cohosh is squaw root. The plant is native to the hillsides of the United States. The herb is only slightly narcotic and sedative. It is anti-spasmodic or useful in relieving spasms, convulsions, etc. It has diaphoretic properties (which result in perspiration). This causes toxic waste to move out through the skin. It moves mucus out through the nose and throat, generally cleansing the system. It is an herb which could, despite opposing interests, become the factor which would enable women, who have hormonal imbalances, the chance to live in harmony with the world and with themselves. If the body does not produce enough of the estrogen hormone, it can cause irregularity of menstrual periods, severe cramps, and emotional nervous problems. We will refer to emotional nervousness because this nervousness is not of the type usually associated with the nervous system, and yet the woman will claim she is extremely nervous. Some women need to take black cohosh each day for two weeks before a period. Some need to take it for the entire month. Other women need take it only a week before the period, and still others need it only for delayed menstrual periods, taking it just a few days before the onset of the period.

Where there is severe cramping, black cohosh will usually stop the cramps within fifteen minutes. (Ginger is also useful for cramps when taken with black cohosh, as it acts as a catalyst to move the herb quickly to the abdominal and pelvic areas.) The problem of how much to take is easily regulated. No woman needs to take more than three 00 size capsules of black cohosh at a time. If three do not solve the problem, it is probable that other glands are involved, and additional related hormone herbs are needed to maintain a balance. Usually one or two 00 size capsules will stop cramps. The exact dosage needed can be observed because when the production of the hormone in the body is adequate, the woman will have a sudden immediate, brief headache from taking black cohosh. When this occurs she will know she has taken too much. The headache is not harmful and does not last. Rather, it seems to be a gauge, similar to insulin shock, but not so severe. Sometimes a woman will stop the estrogen drug and start taking black cohosh and find she cannot take enough without having headaches. In this case again, there are probably other glands involved, and different hormone herbs are needed to create a balance. The change can be made immediately from the drug to black cohosh without any drug withdrawal symptoms.

Lydia Pinkham's formula had fallen into disregard because of the adverse propaganda created by medical science which suggests that anyone who does not use drugs is a quack. Those who stand to lose a great deal economically still fight to maintain control over everyone's health rather than gracefully to allow human need to determine the outcome.

GINSENG FOR THE MAN

Cancer of the *prostate gland* is the most common type of cancer to afflict the American male. This cancer is not uncommon in age bracket 40 — 50 and increases, reaching a high percentage in men of 70 or over. Careful post-mortem studies show that 20% of American men over 60 years old have prostatic cancer. Sometimes when cancer of the prostate in the early stages does not obstruct the flow of urine, it is because the cancer starts at the outer region of the gland and in the beginning does not produce an early impediment of urinary flow. Consequently, prostate cancer is often discovered too late. Hypertrophy, or swelling of the prostate, causes an immediate restriction of urinary flow. This can cause serious damage to the bladder and urether tubes, because of the pressure buildup. Continual pressure can cause serious damage to the kidney tissue resulting in susceptibility to infection. The swelling causes constriction of the urether tubes which go from the bladder through the penis. Where there is no cancer but a continual swelling of the prostate gland, the flow of urine slows down, causing this urine to back up into the bladder, urether tubes, and kidneys. Many other conditions arise, such as skin problems when the body tries to use other organs of elimination to carry off the waste. It is my opinion that often the cause of the swelling is pockets of worms in the lower bowel, causing an irritation and eventual swelling.

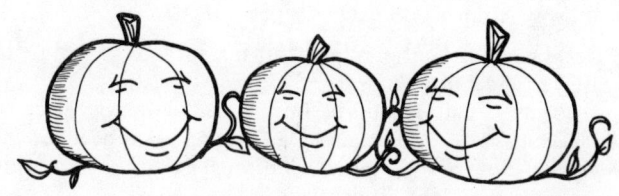

All men over 40 would do well to eat a handful of pumpkin seeds every day as a preventive food. Even when the swelling occurs, pumpkin seed and an herbal laxative will relieve the swelling within 24 hours. A laxative will relieve the pressure fluid build-up until the swelling goes down by draining the fluid from the body to flush the bowels, in this manner relieving the kidneys. Anytime the kidneys, bladder, or prostate are having difficulty performing, the logical solution to relieve the body of waste would be to flush all fluid, or as much as possible, through the bowel until such time as the other organs could again perform. This would, of course, also be necessary with cancer of the prostate when using cancer formulas and corrective diets. There would be a certain amount of laxative in a cancer formula, but probably not enough to relieve the kidneys. Additional laxatives have then been used, but when an herbal laxative (or other kind) is taken on a continual basis, body potassium is also depleted. In these cases it is essential to eat a diet high in vegetables and fruits. Fruits and vegetables are our highest natural sources of potassium. Another good natural source is potassium gluconate. Chemical potassiums made from potash are dangerous and can be given only under a doctor's care.

In cases of prostate cancer, it has been discovered that giving the female hormone or surgical castration alter the growth of the cancer. The administration of the male hormone has an accelerating effect on the growth much as the female estrogen drug has on breast cancer. It has now been made known to the general public that there is great danger in taking estrogen after having a mastectomy or a hysterectomy. When this is done, there can be a reoccurence of the cancer of the breast. Having the fear and knowledge of cancer, the doctor can not conscientiously prescribe the estrogen that her body is no longer producing. With her inability to produce the estrogen necessary to maintain sanity, the woman's problem then becomes mental.

The use of Ginseng as a male hormone acts in a similar way to the drug testosterone which merely gives strength and vigor to the male; and, Ginseng does not have the side effects of testosterone. It would be well for all men over 40 to learn the uses of Ginseng. In the herb world, it is essential to use Ginseng along with any cancer formulas when prostate cancer is present.

The Greeks called Ginseng "plant of the sorcerers" and believed it possessed magical powers.

At night, as if calling out to be noticed, Ginseng gives off a phosphorescent glow. Approaching a Ginseng plant at night causes the flowers to close and the glow is no longer visible. Plant hunters shoot arrows at the plant by daylight.

Ginseng has been used by the Chinese to allay fear and to assist the nervous system. Ginseng increases circulation to the brain, and overcomes nervous prostration and is used as a general tonic. The Chinese believed Ginseng developed character and fortitude as well as a long life; they also believed that it reactivated the sex glands. When this herb has been used for over 5,000 years in China by so many millions of people who have implicit faith in its restorative power, there has to be something Americans have not discovered about Ginseng. Leading medical doctors in China today still look upon Ginseng as a panacea and cure-all, as well as a preventive medicine.

The chief function of a doctor in China was preventive rather than curative. Ginseng is still the most highly regarded and expensive botanical herb in the entire plant kingdom. It increases the vigor of the genital organs and of the gonads in a relationship to longevity.

If Ginseng did not have some psychological effect, its use would have been abandoned a long time ago. In the U.S. we plant and hunt for Ginseng and send thousands of dollars worth of this wonderful herb to China almost with the attitude — that if the superstitious Chinese want to buy this weed we will be glad to gather it for money. While they are asking us to gather it, the Chinese do not tell us much about it, which makes me wonder just who is so smart. Then in turn we buy back their tannic acid tea and drink it with such stupid sophistication as to cause the Chinese to have the last laugh. The export and sale of Ginseng was once a capital crime in China; the use of the plant was kept a guarded secret for thousands of years. When a soldier is wounded or fatigued from battle, the first thing he is given is Ginseng. A powerful antispasmodic, the Chinese give Ginseng for fatigue. Ginseng is also useful in treating reflex nerve diseases, whooping cough, asthma, consumption, fevers, weaknesses of all kinds, and digestion.

GOLDEN SEAL FOR THE DIABETIC

A newspaper article published to raise funds for diabetic research told a young diabetic's story. In it, the young man shared his bitter unhappiness and how he finally had resigned himself to his fate and the daily needle. Near the end of his story, he stated that there is no known cure for diabetes, but merely control of the blood sugar through insulin shots. The concluding paragraphs discussed the climbing numbers of those stricken with diabetes each year, and stated that by 1980, one out of every five individuals could be a diabetic. The author then expressed fear at this prospect and solicited contributions to find the cure that may be just within reach.

When some people, especially children, suddenly become diabetic, in the author's opinion it is because parasites have invaded the islets of Langerhans, and have retarded and then stopped insulin production. When the parasites are removed by herbs such as pumpkin seed or black walnut, normal insulin production will be resumed, if there has been no permanent damage to the glands.

The problems we are having today because of the large consumption of sugar foods are hyperglycemia or hyper-insulinism. These diseases do not occur when there is a problem with insulin production, but rather with constant high acidity caused by sugar in the blood. This condition causes a fault in the mechanism, which results in an over-production of insulin, causing the person to go into a form of insulin shock and then drop down into low blood sugar. Some people experience these highs and lows hourly and daily, making them very difficult people to live with. Often they are almost insane from their own vacillation.

The ability of the body to use sugar is directly related to the individual's hormone balance. Sugar, whether it be black strap sorghum, raw, white, or brown, is still sucrose, and requires sufficient insulin to be changed into glucose before it can be assimilated. This change must be accomplished before reaching the small intestine, where the glucose is absorbed into the bloodstream and used as energy throughout the body. When this change cannot be made effectively, sucrose is spilled out into the urine or absorbed into the blood. The body cannot use sucrose, and this condition causes acidosis, resulting in a coma. Insulin merely allows this change to be accurately accomplished. For the most part, older people who become diabetic do so because they are junk food addicts, and have exhausted the pancreas trying to produce enough insulin to handle the flood of sugar.

During 1964, each person in the United States consumed 95 pounds of sugar. Not only does the public consume much more today, but it also consumes more of the foodless foods associated with sugar: soft drinks, bakery goods, candies, chocolates, jams, jellies, canned goods, gelatin desserts, ice cream, etc. Because we transport and store a large percentage of our food supply, manufacturers feel that it is necessary to preserve foods with chemical additives. Because they need to hide the distasteful chemical bitterness, they use a sugar as a coverup.

As a matter of interest, sugar production is considered one of man's most important industries. Sugar is not only used as a food, but also in the production of nylon, monosodium glutamate, in plasticizers to make plastic tougher, and in carbon paper, phonograph records, many drugs, dyes, cosmetics and even synthetic rubber.

Anytime there is a monetary loss, it will not be taken by big business; rather, it is the average poor citizen who bears the loss. It is he who buys these poisoned sugar commodities, with the thought that someone has so nicely packaged and prepared a wonderful new time-saver for him. When we consider the cost in advertising, packaging, poor food value, poisons in the food which cause sickness and pain, and eventual medical and funeral cost, what have we really saved by allowing these designing men to dictate what we eat?

There are also thousands of pounds of sugar used annually in the tobacco industry. If the use of sugar in edible products alone were cut down, the industry would suffer greatly. Because big business interests refuse to suffer even if the people who buy their products must suffer, brain washing through advertising has reached the point that the average person will say that sugar is one of man's most important foods. Manufacturers give us an early start on the road to diabetes by putting sugar in baby foods and formulas. This distorts the baby's taste, cursing the child with an addiction to sugar from the start.

When the song, "Junk Food Junkie", was played for the first time on a local radio station, the announcer said, "I don't quite understand that song." Anyone who knows about nutrition can easily relate to the song, as they know that deviation from a good diet to junk food yields obvious negative results.

In the *New York Times,* of February 18, 1960, Ezra Taft Benson was quoted as saying: "Lack of knowledge about proper eating was a factor in the weakening of American family life and the rise of juvenile delinquency." The increase of foodless foods has been startling since that time. Are we raising sugarholics, sugar criminals? Are we weakening the structure of family life by this outrageous intake of sugar?

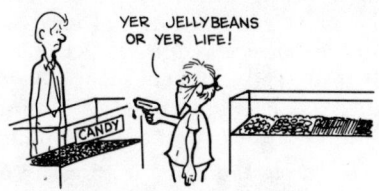

The crime rate in the United States has been related to the rise in sugar consumption, according to J. I. Rodale, in his article, "Does Sugar Make Criminals?" He relates some startling experiences, which I find very easy to believe, since I have observed the same things many times. One set of parents told me that their child would steal to get candy, and after eating large amounts of candy, would become violent to the point of threatening to kill his parents. When they removed sugar, meat and starch from his diet, and fed him vegetables and fruits, he became a totally different, sweet child.

If you are saying, "Sugar gives me a lift and makes me happy, so I will continue to eat it," it may be well to consider its effects on your body and your life. Sugar leeches Vitamin B and calcium from the body, leaving the nervous system shattered. The more sugar used, the more nervous one becomes. The lack of calcium is reflected in hair loss, poor teeth and fingernails, and in osteoporosis, a condition in which bones become porous and soft. The lack of calcium causes brain problems such as senility and stupor, because calcium helps to transport oxygen to the brain. Poor circulation, as well as gland and heart problems, can result from the lack of calcium.

Besides being nearly as addictive as alcohol, sugar can also create a comparable state of acidosis in the body. This condition can cause the person to become argumentative and angry like a drunk, or in some people, cause apparent joviality. Some people may even go into a stupor or become violent. As with alcohol, who can know if large amounts of sugar will produce a criminal or a teddy bear?

Diabetes and Insulin

The philosophy of those who treat diabetes has been to stay completely away from all sugars. However, honey and fruit are not sucrose, but already glucose, and need no insulin to make the change to a usable form. To take a diabetic person completely away from fruit because it contains sugar would be to starve him of the natural glucose he needs to maintain life and energy levels. When a person is taking insulin, he feels (because of the protein theory) that he must eat starches and meats to maintain health. A good hormone balance is required to change starches and meats into the usable form, and when one gland, like the pancreas, is out of balance, other related glands required to bring this balance into proper use do not always perform as they should.

This situation causes the diabetic to easily develop an acidosis condition. The doctor will then give bicarbonate to neutralize the acid caused by inaccurate utilization of meats and starches, and then give needed glucose to maintain life — the life of a diabetic! However, when a diabetic goes on a mild food diet of fruits, vegetables, nuts and seeds (which are mostly glucose), the acids begin to alkalize, causing the burden of the acidosis to be lessened. The diabetic needs to relieve the burden from the glands with a mild food diet. Then, he can add golden seal or juniper berries, the natural hormone herbs which act in the body as natural insulin does. This natural insulin must be used every day when the body is not producing its own. Only small smounts of golden seal and juniper are required when the diabetic is on the mild food diet, unless there is permanent damage to the pancreas. When this has been the case, up to 30 or more capsules a day of golden seal root are required. A small handful of juniper or cedar berries, or six to eight capsules of juniper, are equally effective.

Juniper berries have been used with great success as a diuretic and, like golden seal, act as natural insulin. Here again, a diuretic would seem inconsistent as an insulin. Juniper, however, acts in the same way to correct the mechanism or, where permanent damage has been done, acts in the body as if the body had produced the insulin. Juniper berries, or cedar berries, have the same properties and act equally as well as a natural insulin. There are other special uses for juniper berries which are so specific that the quick action is astounding. Even a serious kidney infection which may have continued for an extended period, can be stopped within a day or two by taking juniper oil — approximately two or three 0 size capsules a day. Kidney pain can be relieved within minutes after chewing a few of the berries.

Juniper, again like golden seal, is antibiotic, and is used both to fumigate a sick room or to gargle with tea or one can chew a few berries after exposure to contagious disease. Juniper has been used as one of the best herbs in the condition of dropsy, for all urinary problems, (bladder, kidney and mucus condition of the bladder, infections, etc.) This remarkable herb has also been used effectively to treat gonorrhea and leucorrhea. Equal parts of uva ursia, clevers and buchu, enhance juniper's ability to draw the fluid of an edema condition from the body. These herbs in combination are useful to relieve fluid trapped anywhere in the body, such as in glycoma or even with water on the knee, swelling in the legs or fluid in the head area. Juniper or cedar berries have the ability to restore the pancreas when there has been no permanent damage.

Finding that golden seal and juniper berries act like insulin is a great discovery, but there are many other important uses for these wonderful herbs. The interesting thing about golden seal, for example, is that not only is it antibiotic but it also has the ability to stop internal bleeding and internal swelling. When golden seal is used instead of insulin, it acts to stop the diabetic hemorrhage that occurs in the vitrus part of the eye which can result in detachment of the retina causing partial blindness. If this hemorrhage occurs too often, complete blindness is the result: therefore in my opinion use of golden seal would be superior to insulin.

Because of the over-acid condition caused in diabetics by the inability to change sucrose sugar to glucose leaving a residue of acid sucrose in the blood, more Vitamin C is required to neutralize these acids, resulting in the apparent lack of Vitamin C, which in turn causes a weakening of the veins and capillaries. Because of this weakness, the capillaries and veins break easily, resulting in blindness or open sores that will not heal.

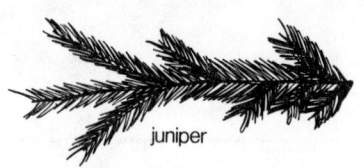
juniper

Because of golden seal's action on internal bleeding, this weakness and breaking can not only be stopped at the onset of hemorrage, but can prevent the diabetic hemorrhage.

When golden seal is used in place of insulin, other advantages can be noticed. It seems that the alkaloid part of golden seal acts as an alkalizer similar to Vitamin C, giving strength to the veins. Golden seal is a diuretic herb also, although this seems inconsistent since the first symptom of diabetes is heavy urination in copious daily amounts. Golden seal somehow has a way of correcting the mechanism which changes sucrose to glucose, (or it is acting as if the body had produced insulin) then with the simulated production of insulin, the body makes the change in the same way it does with insulin. In whatever way this is accomplished, it works.

When golden seal is used for hyperglycemia or hyper-insulinism, caused when there is an excess of insulin rather than a deficiency. (It is as though the pancreas overshoots its mark and produces too much insulin.) would seem inconsistent again to give insulin if the over-production of insulin were the problem. Here again golden seal has a mystical, wonderful power to regulate all systems and prevent the body mechanism from flooding the system with too much insulin when certain foods are ingested.

The Indians of North America taught the settlers how to use golden seal. Golden seal has been used with great success on the mucus membrane. For swelling in the eyes, it can be used as an eye wash and has a soothing effect.

Other Uses for Golden Seal

As we watch with wonder and thanksgiving for the way this herb works, we are continually amazed by its versatility. We have a big white tom cat at our house who has had to fight fiercely to maintain his domain. He had a sore that his opponenets kept tearing open for about a week until my daughter powdered him soundly with a spoonful of dry golden seal while he was asleep. Upon awakening, he stretched and leaned around to give his wound the usual lick. Have you ever seen the look of "yecch" on an animal's face? Well, this was the look he had, and the other cats who kept biting at his wound must have also been discouraged by its bitterness, because within a few days the wound was healed. The next time he had a cut, as soon as he got a whiff of the golden seal, he lay very still and allowed it to be powdered on his wound.

There are many other medicinal uses for golden seal. It has been used for inflamed eyes and sores in the mouth. When used with myrrh for pyorrhea, it has no equal. This herb has been used for skin disorders, acne and eczema, and for stomach and liver problems. Golden seal, mixed equal parts of eyebright and bayberry and used as an eye wash, will remove some superficial cataracts from the surface of the eyes. Golden seal exercises a considerable influence on the nervous system and has been used in conjunction with cayenne for chronic alcoholism. When the stomach is over-acid or unable to empty, golden seal acts immediately to neutralize the acids and empty the stomach. In days past, it was considered one of the best bitter tonic herbs (called the "bitters") and was used for digestion. When mixed with myrrh, ½ part, echinacea, ½ part, and 1 part golden seal, then used as a wash or douche for leucorrhea, eczema or sore throat, these herbs have an influence superior to any other agents.

Golden seal is unsurpassed in its many uses and is sometimes called the "cure-all" herb. People who have used and believe in golden seal have not convinced themselves about it without reason. When I was lecturing in San Bernadino, a woman gave her story about golden seal. She said she was in charge of a half-way house for heroin addicts. After reading my book, *Is Any Sick Among You,* she began to give them golden seal and licorice and discovered that the heroin would be out of their bodies within four days. These people were so thrilled with the results, the State of California was approached for funds to pay for herbs and they were granted the money. However, I heard of a report that some addicts were using Golden Seal to erase traces in the urine after taking heroin when they have been cheating while away from the half-way house. I was sorry to hear such a report.

KELP FOR GLANDULAR BALANCE

Iodine is essential to the restoration of the pituitary, adrenal, pineal, thyroid, and parathyroid glands. The only way to restore glandular balance is to assist the over-worked gland by cleaning the body and by administering the relative hormone herbs — which acts in the body as if the body had produced the needed hormones.

The activities of the thyroid have to do with the metabolism of protein, carbohydrate, and fat, regulation of sodium and potassium, retention of fluid, as well as growth, the nervous system, muscles, the circulatory system, and the endocrine glands. Some people are given the thyroid drug to lose weight in an attempt to reverse their bodies from being underactive to overactive so as to burn off the fat. Some people are given radioactive treatment to stop the over-production. Since kelp or dulse iodine works well in either case, I cannot help but believe they are completely off the track when it comes to treatment of the thyroid. The medical manuals and books on the thyroid seem to be a mass of confused contradictions.

The thyroid gland seems to be low in iodine when the body is undergoing a toxic contagion, a cold, and also in chronic disease. This gland often has a related attachment to any of the other glands malfunctioning, but sometimes its problems are singular. When swelling of the throat occurs, as in goiter, the gland is more active at this time, and the iodine content is lower. It has been taught that when iodine is taken by mouth, a considerable portion is taken up by the thyroid: the thyroid promptly takes back most of the iodine, sort of a recycling process.

The body practices such great economy with respect to iodine, utilizing the bulk of its store repeatedly in the hormone synthesis of iodine derived from the daily breakdown, that only a fraction is excreted; 0.2 milligrams — seven times this amount — is required for hormone production. With this information in mind, it would indicate that swelling or infection caused by toxic waste increases the need for iodine, also increasing the amount being sent out into circulation to kill the bacteria living in such waste. If the iodine were used up, rendering it unable to be recycled, it would show up on the basic metabolic rate (B.M.R.) as being lowered.

When the thyroid does not produce enough iodine to perform its functions, and too much waste is added to the body, the thyroid works in a way we could call active, like whipping a tired horse, into the swelling condition we call goiter. Kelp or dulse iodine can be used for what is termed hypo or hyper-thyroid (inactive or overactive) with the result of glandular improvement. This is not the case with the thyroid drug.

The first iodine ash was made from seaweed or kelp and was discovered by a French chemist, Bernard Courtois, in 1811. In 1814 another French chemist, Joseph Louis Gay-Lussac proved it was a chemical element. Sir Humphrey Davy named the element iodine from the Greek word (ioeides) which means violets colored, since the ash obtained is a violet color.

Iodine has found many uses in chemistry, for the most part as an antiseptic. A solution of iodine mixed with alcohol is called tincture of iodine, and is used on cuts and infections, ringworms, sore throat, etc. While the human body requires this important trace mineral for proper growth, chemical iodines are poison when taken internally in large amounts. Naturalists who use kelp in its whole state find it to be helpful for infections, colds and flu, as well as in maintaining general well-being.

When there is a lack of iodine, such as would whip the tired horse even further, a state we call cretin or myxedema results. The cretin or myxedema victim further proves my theory by his being unable to combat acute disease. These people always have a cold, constipation, respiratory problems, etc. They will die at a very young age in cretinism, and soon in cases of myxedema, if something is not done. It is well known that an inadequate hormone production of the thyroid causes cretin condition during fetal or early life, and a myxedema condition at any time in life, but it is not known why. The glands of the thyroid and neck can harden from too much mucus waste in the body, from a cement-like mucus in the entire area causing related ear trouble. Swelling glands can also force the vertebrae in the neck to move and pinch nerves, thus creating other problems. The bowels and the heart can be affected also. If this mucus remains too long, it may lead to a cancerous condition. Myxedema can result when there has been a removal of the thyroid: the person rapidly develops the appearance of a cretin. Severe myxedema may cause wasting rather than obesity, a state of cachexia as in malignancies.

There are two tests to determine the activity of the thyroid: B.M.R. (basic metabolism rate) and P.B.I. (protein bound iodine). In the case of hypo-active thyroid (under), the symptoms are goiter, cretinism, myxedema, and obesity. The B.M.R., would show normal or low, and the P.B.I. would be low. The treatment used in the medical world would be iodine. The symptoms with hyper (over-active) active thyroid would be high pulse, hypertension, protrusion of the eyeballs, arterial fibrillation, and apathy, with often an enlarged heart. Older persons may be apathetic, with heart failure. Wasting can also occur, and the P.B.I. would show high, the medical treatment usually being surgical removal of part of the gland to reduce activity or any tumor. A new treatment, the use of radioactive iodine, theorizes that if the gland is producing too much iodine, radioactive iodine will pick it up, possibly destroying part of the gland. What then happens to all that radioactivity? The thyroid becomes weakened and functions either over- or under-actively because of too much mucus waste, when it either gives up or over-produces. When the body keeps increasing the toxic body waste, calling for more iodine, the thyroid can swing either way, as I see it, depending on its ability to produce hormone.

Just because only a small amount of iodine is excreted does not necessarily mean that iodine is recycled as it is used; it could be used up completely. Where there is an over-production caused by the necessity to combat bacteria (too much mucus), the over-production could have an effect like that of taking iodine poison. When the correct amount is sent forth into the body, it could have the positive effect of killing germs like painting iodine on a wound. The tonsil secretes iodine, killing the bacteria as it enters the mouth; and when we remove the tonsil, we remove the body's helpful insurance against invading bacteria.

Among people who search for natural methods of healing, kelp

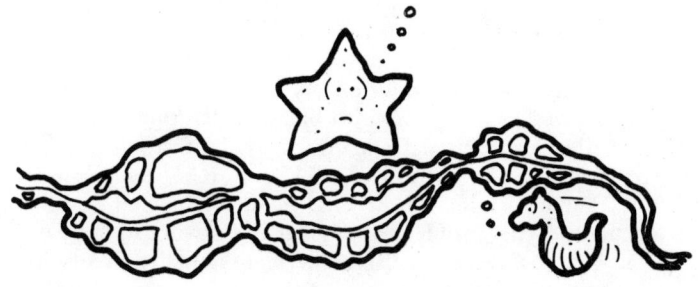

has become well-known as an herb full of minerals and primarily rich in iodine. The kelp plant is seen on all beaches, but the largest kelp beds are off the coast of Ireland, Scotland, and England. Masses of giant kelp also grows in the Pacific waters off the coast of North and South America. The amounts of iodine obtained from four to 15 pounds per ton. Kelp contains common salt, sodium carbonate, sodium and potassium sulfates, and potassium and sodium iodides in a natural plant form.

Alkaline ash is made by burning the seaweed. The crude alkali obtained from the ash was once used to obtain the alkalies for soaps. Kelp is also dried and used in many fertilizers. However, kelp is used among natural food circles in its whole state to increase the mineral content of the body, particularly that of iodine. Pure potassium iodide taken from potash potassium is a bluish-black crystalline solid which will unite with metals such as potassium to form salts of iodine used in medicines, photography and in germicides.

In a lack or overabundance of iodine, a nervous condition is manifest. Iodine is also used with potassium gluconate (a natural potassium) to remove excess fluid from the body. Black walnut is also a high source of iodine. People who live in the goiter belt have wondered why God did not provide iodine for them. They have been provided, however, with a source which grows all over the goiter belt area: on the hull of the black walnut, as well as in the leaf. A strong substance on the hull can cause the hands to break out. The leaf is sold by many herb companies in powder form and is milder but is still a high, rich source of natural iodine.

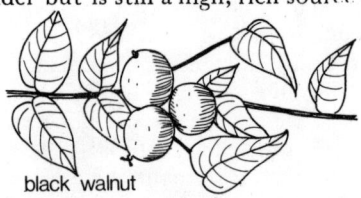
black walnut

LICORICE FOR HYPOGLYCEMIA

We have coined a new word we call hypoglycemia. A product of our age, this word had to come into being to describe adrenal exhaustion we develop, caused from the stress of a fast moving society in combination with a stress diet of high starch, protein, sugars and a low intake of minerals. Because medical science has called this particular adrenal problem hypoglycemia, I will use this word also to explain the use of licorice. There are actually two types, hyper and hypo, hyper having to do with the pancreas as well as the adrenals.

Hypoglycemia is a malfunction of the adrenal glands. The adrenal cortex has two parts: the medulla, which secretes the hormone adrenalin, allowing us to fight or run in emergency; and the cortex, which secretes the hormone cortin. This hormone allows us to stand daily stress and worry. There are other hormones which have been found in the adrenal glands, but we will discuss only these two.

In hypoglycemia, sugar is taken to give a stimulating lift in the hope of overcoming depression, but the problem is thereby compounded, as sugar leaches the Vitamin B and the calcium from the body causing more stress, losing more potassium and body tone. The insulin is raised to an unnatural high to take care of the sugar, somehow extending past its needs and afterwards dropping to a new low, causing a low blood sugar called insulin shock (overdose of insulin). Immediately we add sugar to lift us up again, and a vicious circle has begun. Having found the herbs that act like cortisone (cortin hormone) to be helpful in this case, I feel it is important for me to make it known. To begin, a brief history about cortisone may be of interest.

With the help of the African Witch Doctor, the seeds of the plant strophanthus were used to make cortisone or Compound E. Because of the rain forest and difficulty in harvesting this plant, cortisone was later made from the Mexican wild yam. Cortisone was made synthetically. When the adrenal glands begin to break down from too much stress (sometimes a shock, too much worry, or too much sugar eaten) hypoglycemia or Addison's Disease develops.

Addison's Disease is characterized by symptoms similar to hypoglycemia, with the addition that Addison's Disease becomes terminal. According to medical standards, the following are some of the symptoms: blotchy pigment on large parts of the body, an intolerance to heat or cold develops, there is a reduction in capacity for muscular work, with weakness, inability to stand any negative or positive stress or emotional excitement. Sometimes resulting in nervous breakdown or even insanity, complete exhaustion, a feeling one is going to die, the inability to digest food. When the cortin hormone is not produced at all, the body dies as with lack of insulin. The absence of cortin can also result, prior to Addison's Disease, in arthritis. The giving of cortisone for arthritis is a help only when adrenal malfunction is the cause. When the cause is years of incorrect eating, cortisone is worthless; but doctors did continue to give it for many ailments, in the hope that some other disease would respond to the new wonder drug. Medical doctors have discovered that cortisone helps in treatment of some skin disease; but here again, the skin problem was probably related to the stress factor involving the adrenals. If a natural herb-like cortisone is used instead, the complications, side effects, and disillusionment that come from using the synthetic drug can be avoided.

At one time in my life I felt I had an edge on all truth. I had studied diet and health, taught exercise, even had my own women's gym. I had fasted frequently and raised organic gardens. Then a shocking, traumatic, painful grief that I could not surmount came into my life. Within one year and a half, I had developed Addison's Disease. Knowing what I did about the body and about cortisone (that life expectancy is only about ten years when taking this drug), I prayed to find a way to save my life. I knew I must take cortisone or die, but felt there must be an herb which would act the same as cortisone. I received a blessing and was blessed that I would find the answer to my problem. Three days later, I found it — licorice.

licorice

Licorice is of the pea family and is a perennial herb with roots which grow very deep into the ground. The root contains a wealth of healing, medicinal properties as well as a valuable flavoring. It is native to Southern Europe, Asia Minor, Russia, Spain, Iraq, Turkey and British East Africa, with only negligible quantities of this herb coming from other countries. There is a substance known as glycyrrhizic acid in the root which makes the herb sweeter than sugar by about fifty times, and also sweeter than saccharin. All other sweets cause an increased thirst, whereas licorice has the ability to allay thirst.

Because of its sweet taste and good flavor, it has been used to disguise disagreeable flavors in medicines and has been used to flavor cigars, cigarettes, candy, gum, and ice cream. After the flavor is extracted, the remaining fibers are used to make fire fighting foam, box board, insulation board, and other products. Each year the United States imports vast quantities of the root and liquid extract. Licorice was used in ancient Greece and Rome for colds, coughs, and sore throat. It was believed by ancient Hindus to increase sexual vigor and was long maintained by the Chinese for strength and endurance.

As I began to experiment with it, I found that if I took two 00-size capsules of powdered licorice root a day. I could go twenty-four hours. As soon as twenty-four hours were up, I would go back to feeling the same way. You may say, "Well, then, it must be addictive." So is eating. Like insulin, cortin must be replaced when it is used up. I learned as my body healed, however, that when I lived on fruit only, licorice was not necessary. At first, the problems attached to adrenal malfunction would not allow fruit diets, or fasting. (The vitamins and herbs necessary to restore, so as to be able to use more fruits, are listed in the chapters on herbs and home remedies.) You can stop taking licorice without going into shock, unlike what would happen if you suddenly stopped taking cortisone. The spirit whispers many things; we must learn to listen.

Licorice acts like a steroid. Cortisone is a steroid sugar. Licorice does not, however, bring the high insulin reaction that sugar does. For a while, the hypoglycemic must remain on the ups and downs he has become used to until he can regulate the insulin-type herbs to the cortisone-type herbs. To clarify this, let me say that I believe it is the taking of sugar (sucrose) which brings on the shock associated with low blood sugar. Adding a little golden seal when taking too much sugar assists the body in its use. Golden seal acts somewhat like insulin but does not increase the insulin to a shock rate, yet rather somehow assists the body in the use of the sugar. Then to add something comparable to cortin (adrenal hormone), licorice can be used as a steroid. Licorice gives a better lift than sugar, without increasing the blood sugar demand for insulin and bringing on the shock. As I see it, the greatest enemy to the hypoglycemic person is sugar, but not the natural fruit sugars their bodies so desperately need.

When people who have been under severe stress, overworking the adrenals and becoming extremely nervous and irritable, begin to take licorice, they think they have suddenly, spiritually, arrived. Many who suffer in mental institutions could be helped with this wonderful herb.

We can see now why soldiers could stand the stress of war while using licorice and why it was believed to have such strengthening powers. When the adrenals are exhausted, every daily task becomes a mountain. Fatigue and depression become our middle name. When we take licorice under these circumstances, our whole attitude changes, and we suddenly have strength and energy and can cope with daily stress and worry. Like a miracle, our whole attitude changes from near insanity to peaceful calm, without any of the doped out sensations of tranquilizers and drugs. Those who have learned and experienced this are grateful for the wondrous properties God has placed in this blessed root.

History records that licorice was used by the soldiers of Alexander and carried on their person the way our soldiers carried penicillin. It was used to allay thirst during the desert fighting and marching in the Middle East. As a medicine it has persisted for more than 4,000 years. Aside from all the many uses, both ancient and modern, where licorice has blessed the world, may I teach you still another entirely new concept of its great value? We are only beginning to glimpse the potential service to humanity that this amazing herb has to offer. In all ages past, licorice has been treated with the utmost respect not knowing why it gave us its blessing of strength, vigor and as the Chinese believed, "warded off old age."

Pliny said: "The juice of Liquirice reduced to thick consistense if it were put under the tongue is singular for to cleare the voice, and therewith, both thirst and hunger may be slaked and allaied."

Nicholas Culpepper wrote: "Liqorice root, boiled in water with some maidenhair and figs, makes a good drink for those who have a dry cough or hoarseness, wheezing or shortness of breath... It is also a cleansing agent, and at the same time softening and soothing, and therefore balsamic.

"The juice, or extract, is made by boiling the fresh roots in water, straining the decoction, and when the impurities have settled, evaporating it over a gentle heat until it will no longer stick to the fingers. It is better to cut the roots into small pieces before boiling them, as the healing agencies in the root will by that means be better extracted. A pound of liquorice root boiled in three pints down to one quart will be found the best for all purposes."

"The juice of the liquorice root is most effective, and may be obtained by squeezing the roots between two rollers. When made with due care, it is exceedingly sweet and of a much more agreeable taste than the root itself."

Licorice must have been a favorite of the Egyptian Pharaohs, because so much has been found in the tombs and because it is still used as a beverage in Egypt today.

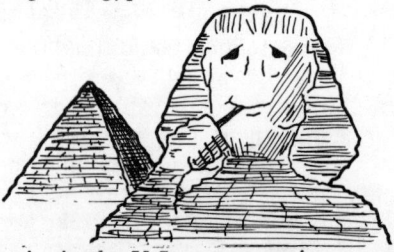

The drug industries in the U.S. use a certain amount of the large quantities of licorice imported, because of the demulcent and expectorant properties, such as in the preparation of pills in coatings, etc. Most of the vast supply of licorice, however, is used by tobacco industries for flavoring. Some is also used as a fertilizer for mushrooms. The Chinese also use licorice in soy sauce. In England, licorice is used in cough syrups, cough drops, ale, and beer. In France and Belgium, steel workers drink a licorice beverage in place of water.

The 17th edition of the U.S. Dispensatory states: "Liquorice is a useful demulcent, much employed in cough mixtures, and frequently added to infusions or decoctions in order to cover the taste or obtund the acrimony of the principle medicine. A piece of it held in the mouth and allowed to dissolve slowly is often found to allay cough by sheathing the irritated membrane..."

According to the *Science Digest,* 1950, licorice has female hormonal properties. You can ask any grandmother over 70 years old and she will tell you that licorice has been used for its laxative effect.

LOBELIA FOR RESTORING THE SICK

Lobelia is one of the greats in the herb world. Anyone who knows about herbs is aware of the marvelous possibilities of this herb, both in formula or by itself. Lobelia is the best relaxant in the herb kingdom. For asthma, emphysema, TB, nervous disorder, withdrawal from drugs, it is without exception the best herb available.

Priddy Meeks, the Mormon pioneer Herbalist and Thomsonian practitioner, was enthusiastic in his praise of this great herb, after using it almost a half-century in medical practice:

> "I sometimes look upon Lobelia as being Super-natural, although I have been using it for forty-six (46) years. I do not know the extent of its powers and virtues in restoring the sick and at the same time perfectly harmless. Oh! glorious medicine!"

Lobelia will act on the system in complete conformity with the laws of health. When there are obstructions caused by broken health laws and the body then fails to function as nature intends, Lobelia will remove those obstructions wherever they are located. Lobelia will permeate the whole system till it finds where the obstruction is seated, and there it will spend its influence and powers by relaxing the parts obstructed. One should always accompany lobelia with cayenne pepper, which is the purest and best stimulant that is known in the compass of medicine. It will increase the very life and vitality of the system and give the blood a greater velocity and power. When the system is relaxed with lobelia and the blood is stimulated with such power, the combination will act on the whole system. It will act on the whole system like an increased flow of water turned into a muddy spring of water — it will soon run clear.

Lobelia is undoubtedly the best and purest relaxant in the field of herbal medicine. That is the reason lobelia is so good in child bed cases. It puts the system exactly in the situation the laws of nature would have it be to perform that object. Those in the habit of using lobelia in such cases look forward in pleasing anticipation of having a good time without the forebodings of trouble so common to women.

Samuel Thomson was the discoverer of lobelia. He said of the use of lobelia:

> "I have seen some lie and sob like a child that has been punished for two hours, not able to speak or raise their hands, to use their head and the next day be about and soon get well."

> "In cases where they have taken considerable opium and this medicine (lobelia) is administered, it will in its operation, produce the same appearance and symptoms that are produced by opium when first given, which having lain dormant, is roused into action by the enlivening qualities of this medicine and the patient will often be thrown into a senseless state: The whole system will be one complete mass of confusion, tumbling in every direction, and it will take two or three to hold them on the bed. Sometimes they grow cold as though dying; remaining in this way from two to eight hours, and then awake, like one from sleep, after a good night's rest, entirely calm and sensible as though nothing ailed them. It is seldom they ever have more than one of these turns; as it is the last struggle of the disease and they gradually begin to recover from that time."

The FDA has recently tried to stop the sale of Lobelia, labeling it as poisonous. This labeling recalls the following incident recorded by Jethro Kloss in *Back to Eden:*

> Samuel Thomson employed lobelia quite extensively in Vermont, New York, New Hampshire, and Massachusetts as early as 1795. There are extant many allopathic works such as Thatcher's Dispensatory (1817), the U.S. Dispensatory, Griffith, Royle, Carson, etc.; wherein the reader is informed that "Thomson himself was tried for murder for killing a man with this article."

> Did one know nothing outside the medical records, one would possibly accept the conclusion that Thomson was a careless empiric, who was called to account for using a deadly article.

We give the student a concise outline of the facts of the case. The trial took place in December, 1809, before the Supreme Court in Salem, Mass. Thomson was charged with the murder of one Ezra Lovett, Jr., by the administering of lobelia. The complaint was laid by a Dr. French, an allopathic physician, who had repeatedly persecuted Thomson. So bitterly had this Dr. French persecuted Thomson that the latter had been compelled to take steps to have Dr. French bound over to keep the peace, because the M.D. had publicly threatened to blow Thomson's brains out.

Following this incident, Dr. French, seeking an opportunity to injure this wonderful man, Thomson, finally procured Thomson's arrest on a charge of murder. (It is evidently the vemon of French and his charge against Thomson, that is the basis of the allopathic claim that lobelia is a poison.) We quote a few lines from Dr. Thomson's report of the case: "Just before night, Dr. French arrived with the sheriff and ordered me to be delivered by the constable to the sheriff. Dr. French again vented his spleen upon me by the most savage abuse that language could express saying that I was a murderer, that I had murdered fifty and he could prove it, that I should be either hung or sent to the State Prison for life, and he would do all in his power to have me convicted.

I was then put in irons by the sheriff, and conveyed to the jail in Newburyport and confined in a dungeon with a man who had been convicted of an assault upon a girl six years of age. I was not allowed a chair or a table, nothing but a miserable straw bunk on the floor, with one poor blanket which had never been washed. I was put into this prison on the tenth day of November, 1809." He then tells of the colds, the filth, the vermin that infested the place, etc.

As there was no session of the court until the fall of the next year, it was expected that he would have to lie in this unhealthy confinement for a year, which would most likely have killed him. There were, however, some eminent friends who had benefited from his work, who, through their influence, after making fifteen trips from Salem to Boston, secured a hearing before Judge Parsons in a special session on December 10, 1809.

Vol. VI, Massachusetts Criminal Reports, contains the report of the trial written by Judge Parsons himself. It is supposed that the Judge was favorably disposed to the prosecution, and gave only that which plain justice called for to Thomson. The report states, among other things, Thomson, "had administered the like medicines with those given to the deceased to several of his patients, who had died under his hands." This charge was made by the Solicitor General; and to prove this statement, he called several witnesses of whom but one appeared. He testified that he had been the prisoner's patient for an "oppression at his stomach," that he took the emetic powders several times in three or four days and was relieved from his complaint, which had not since returned, and there was no evidence in the case that the prisoner in the course of his very novel practice had experienced any fatal accident among his patients.

"As the court was satisfied that the evidence produced by the commonwealth did not support the indictment, the prisoner was put upon his defense. The prisoner was acquitted."

Such is the report of the case (written by the Judge himself) that evidently gave rise to the blind repetition that lobelia is a poison. There were justices on the bench at the trial, and only the blindness of allopathic prejudices continues to ban from general use one of our best remedies.

After this time, laws were sought forbidding the prescribing, selling, or even the giving away of lobelia; meanwhile the same brand of allopathic knave went on prescribing arsenic, antimony, strychnine, prussic acid, etc. During the following years, many of the reformatory physicians were prosecuted and allopath regulars swore on oath that ten, eight, or even four grains of lobelia were sufficient to cause death. Yet no proof was ever found that any life had ever been lost or injured by it, while some physicians and many patients testified that they had taken from half an ounce upwards in the space of a few hours, always to their benefit.

Back to Eden by Jethro Kloss

SAFFRON FOR DIGESTION AND STIFFNESS

The Bible mentions saffron among the chief spices: "Thy plants are an orchard of pomegranates, with pleasant fruits; camphire, with spikenard. Spikenard and saffron; calamus and cinnamon, with all trees of frankincense, myrrh and aloes, with all the chief spices." *Song of Solomon* 4:13-14.

Saffron has been used for centuries to make a brilliant yellow dye. It has also been used as an aromatic food flavoring and to color candy. The flavor of saffron is used as a seasoning especially among people living in Europe and India.

About 4,000 flowers will yield approximately one ounce of commercial saffron. It is produced from the purple autumn crocus by drying the stigmas and part of the stylus of the flower. The odor is sweet and the flavor is bitter-sweet, not at all unpleasant to the taste.

William Salmon in his family dictionary (in 1644) said, regarding saffron, that it was good for yellow jaundice and rheumatism. He added that if it was used with wine, the person would not become drunk and that it would also heal bites of serpents and spiders.

Henry Burdon (1734) said in his book, *The Fountain of Youth*, that saffron corrects acidity of the stomach.

William Cockburn (1669), in his book, *Account of Nature*, said it was useful for dysentery.

B. Frank School, in a later book written in 1925, said saffron was used for rheumatism, measles and scarlet fever, and that it causes sweating.

Equal parts of catnip and saffron have been used with excellent results for scarlet fever. The reason it was useful for fever is that it causes profuse perspiration when taken hot and causes the skin to break out, if — as in the case of a childhood disease — there is high fever, as in measles. As soon as the break-out occurs, the fever goes down and relief from the pain is on the way.

Medical Research

Medical doctors discovered that the uric acid build-up in a gout patient could be relieved by a drug called *colchicine* made from *meadow saffron roots*. The remarkable result from its use relieved acute gout pain, but did not help any other form of arthritis. *Gout* is a disease known in the history books of antiquity as the plague and misery of kings and wealthy prominent men. The disease is due to a defect in the body chemistry (according to the medical books) where too much oil in the diet causes the chalky salts of uric acid. The kidneys normally excrete uric acid from the body, but in the gouty person they do not do so efficiently and cannot excrete in balance to production. The use of too much oil in the diet could be the cause of the body's inability to carry off the over-production, but it is my opinion that the cause stems from a beginning imbalance in the adrenal glands. It is interesting to note that an attack of acute gout can be brought on by several forms of stimuli — emotional stress, marital troubles, quarrels, surgery, and certain drugs, such as liver injections. Therefore, it would be reasonable to suspect that an over-stressful situation causing fatigue of the adrenals could be the beginning cause of the uric acid build-up.

It may also be interesting to note that an obese person losing weight too fast can become gouty because of the overload of fat being eliminated by the body, resulting in the build-up of uric acid. The normal treatment of gout would be the prescription drugs *colchicine* or *phenylbutazone,* which drugs may promptly cause nausea, vomiting, and diarrhea. The physician will then reduce the dosage. Relief comes because the uric acids are drawn off through other routes of elimination.

Symptoms of gout are manifested by pain in the big toe, but other joints are also eventually affected. Meat seems to be a great enemy of the gouty person, as it builds uric acid faster than anything but oil. Even with the use of gout drugs to control and help in acute attacks, formation of *urate deposits* begin slowly to accumulate. The end result of such accumulation is eventually kidney stones. Then prescription drugs such as *probeneciad* and *sulfapyrazone* are used to flush fluids. At this point the disease has become chronic. It is also interesting that using aspirin for pain will *nullify* the effects of the uricosuric drugs, causing a further retention of uric acid.

Saffron does not neutralize uric acid; it merely allows the person to use oil, stopping the build-up of uric acid. Where there is also a need to draw off uric acid the way certain *uricosuric* drugs do, dandelion is then the herb to use. Dandelion flushes or draws off such uric acids as have already been built up in the body prior to the use of saffron. It can now be readily seen how saffron could be a wonderful preventative for kidney stones in people prone to such a condition.

Why Saffron Helps

To help in the understanding of why saffron works on these cases, it must also be explained that this sort of uric acid is building up around the joints and holds calcium in deposit in an arthritic person. Nevertheless it all goes back to the adrenals' inability to produce enough cortin hormone to stand daily stress and worry. It is my opinion — without going into details on the subject of adrenals — that the reason saffron works on such gouty cases, and is also helpful in adrenal cortial malfunction, is that it acts almost as a hormone in such a way as to allow the body to use oil, where the body otherwise would build up uric acid.

Also, when a person has hypoglycemia or adrenal fatigue and the body is not producing enough cortin hormone, the body builds up lactic acid. Lactic acid is the end product of over-exercise, and stiffness and soreness are its results. The usual route for lactic acid is that it returns to the liver and is changed to glycogen, to be used later for energy, but when the adrenals do not produce enough cortin, this process is stopped and the lactic acid remains in the tissues. Eventually it seeps into the abdominal cavity and stomach, interfering with digestion and causing a burning acid stomach. Saffron in some wonderful way stops the lactic acid build-up.

If a person has a lot of yard work or exercise to do early in the spring when certain muscles have not been used all winter, taking saffron before the work day will be an amazing experience, because no stiffness or soreness will be felt. Saffron will also neutralize the acid stomach caused when certain types of hypoglycemic persons eat fruit. A person who is subject to gout or kidney stones can even eat oil and meat as long as he takes saffron with each meal that includes meats or oils.

YUCCA FOR ARTHRITIS

Yucca belongs to the agave family. The shrub grows in such a way to have a striking and beautiful appearance and many people in the southern California area plant them as a main attraction in a well decorated yard. As it grows, the yucca becomes a shrub tree and is evergreen and will not shed its leaves annually. Like many desert plants, it will wither some outside leaves.

Botanists and technicians recently seem to be doing intensive studies with this plant because of its known beneficial effects on other desert plants growing around the Yucca. *Let's Live* magazine quotes John W. Yale: "I became fascinated with the idea of these desert plants not only surviving, but actually thriving in this incredible environment — the extreme heat, then extreme cold, absolutely no water for long periods of time and then too much water following sudden cloudbursts," he said. "First, we found that steroid saponin compounds were in high concentration in many of the desert succulents and also in high concentrations in the desert soil itself. We discovered in studying the Yucca that when its leaves died, they slowly disintegrated into a fine dust which then floated through the air. You could actually stand 100 yards down wind from the plant, have some one shake it and you would taste the dust as it hit you." "It became obvious to us," he said, "that the yuccas, and other succulents to a lesser degree, were actually treating large areas of desert around themselves as part of nature's overall survival mechanism." Thus the yucca is acting as a combination wetting and anti-stress agent which helps plants utilize or take up available water.

Yucca Extracts

It has been discovered that an extract from Yucca, called *saponins*, accelerates the organic waste breakdown by microscopic bacteria, so it was used in experiments with waste disposal plants. There was great success with its use and it is still being used in sewage treatment plants in the United States and Canada. It is also used with much success as a cleaning agent. With the use of *sapoin,* a derivative of the Yucca plant, some interesting charts and test cases have resulted. (Tests conducted by Robert Bingham, M.D.; Bernard A. Bellew, M.D.; and Joeva G. Bellew can be found in *The Journal of Applied Nutrition* Vol. 27, No. 2,3.)

It has been found that the yucca plant saponin is a steroid which is *not absorbed* by the intestines in the way that some animal steroids are usable in the body. Some of the reports and findings of their research has been published in *Let's Live* magazine, February, 1975, and again in August, 1975. When some of their testing on arthritics was completed, it was reported that 60.7 percent of the patients who had been given Yucca over a period of one year said they felt less swelling, less pain and stiffness and that 39.3 percent felt no improvement.

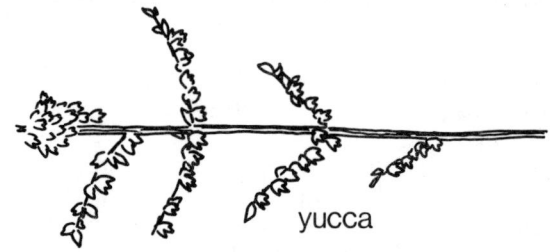

yucca

During this course of study, some interesting information has emerged which could be the clue to why some people are helped with the taking of Yucca. A soap-like material, Yucca will actually lather like soap because it holds large quantities of water within the plant just the way soap holds water against the skin. This is why the yucca can be used as a soap. Testing further reveals it to be a hormonal material, a steroid. The adrenal hormone, *cortisone* is a steroid but the Yucca has a definite action upon the intestinal bacteria, or intestinal flora, living within the human intestines, which actually helps with the digestion of food and prevents certain types of harmful bacteria from flourishing which could cause sickness if too many are accumulated.

Bacterial-intestinal flora are called "friendly bacteria" and are produced by the body itself in a similar way that antibodies are produced. This is similar to the action of a septic tank or the action of organic compost where the friendly red worms, lime, etc., overpower the putrefaction and change what could otherwise be stinking garbage, to a sweet smelling humas. It has been found by its action, that Yucca saponin somehow improves digestion and reduces the tendency to develop accumulations of undigested toxic waste which decompose in the colon, producing foul smelling gases. When a condition is found where such putrefaction exists, it becomes a fertile field for many parasites and many obnoxious worms and bacteria. Disease follows quickly when this situation occurs.

Without the sweetening effect or distraction of unfriendly bacteria by the friendly bacteria, an inability to digest food begins, and the filth of toxic waste begins to invade the entire body through the lymphatic system. As the retention of waste continues, bacteria and parasites increase until the body becomes overwhelmed by such waste to the point that chronic diseases, such as arthritis and cancer merely become manifestations of filth within.

In an attempt to find a use for Yucca in the treatment of arthritis, because it has been discovered to be a steroid (and finding that it cannot be used as a steroid because it does not absorb), researchers may have found another important help to certain types of arthritis in the discovery of a plant B6. If they understood that licorice acts as a steroid for the adrenals, further scientific studies might result in help for more and difficult types of arthritics than they thus far have helped.

There are a number of varieties of the Yucca plant, some grow short while others grow tall with woody scaly trunks. When the plant blossoms, the flowers are shaped like bells. Some varieties have whitish-green flowers. The flowers grow forth from a stem, springing from the center of the clustered leaves. The flowers open at night and give forth a strong fragrance. The Yucca also produces a fruit that may be fleshy or dry, containing many small flat black seeds.

Yucca has a thick tuberous root which spreads as it grows into many tuberous heads. From these tuberous heads the leaves of a long hard texture shoot forth tightly closed together at the bottom, and grey-green in color. The leaves are sharp at the tip and have a hard thread running through them which, when the plant withers, becomes pliant so that it can be used like a rope or string to bind things together. The Yucca plant grows in the West Indies, Virginia, New England, Nevada, California and Arizona, Southern and Southwestern United States. They also grow in the Mexican desert highlands and plateaus. There is a national monument in California named after one of the yucca species called The Joshua Tree Monument containing an important collection of many Yucca species. The popular Northern species is called Adams Needle (*filamentosa*). The Soup Weed (*glauca*) variety is found in the Dakotas and New Mexico.

Nicholas Culpepper says, "The raw juice is dangerous, if not deadly, and it is supposed the Indians poisoned the heads of their darts therewith.' The facts contradict this statement.

The Indians used yucca plants for many useful things. They made sandals, rope, maps, baskets, etc. They ate the flowers raw or cooked. They dried the fleshy fruit for winter and make a drink fermented from the fruit. They even used the plant for their needles and thread, and made soap from the roots and stems. Primitive Indians living in desert areas have used Yucca as a major food source, proven safe by countless generations.

CONDIMENT HERBS

Often when a family begins to change their diet to include more vegetables and fruit and less starch and meats, it becomes a real problem for the mother to get her family to eat the vegetables. When mother learns to cook vegetables properly with herbs, she can then become a gourmet cook, and her meal becomes an exotic experience for her family.

To enhance the taste of vegetables suitable even to a person who lives mostly on raw food and whose body is very clean internally, minimum cooking is essential. Cooking should be done in stainless steel with a low heat to maintain vitamin and mineral values as well as aroma and taste. The vegetable should be cooked, but only until slightly tender, as in the Chinese manner of cooking. Some vegetables need only to be barely warmed. Remove the pan from the flame and add soft, cold-pressed oil and condiment herbs. The herbs are never cooked but the pan steaming will bring out their flavor and aroma. As one begins to experiment with different tastes in herbs, one should begin lightly as it is difficult to correct overseasoning but always easy to add more. Learn to limit the number of herb dishes you serve — only one herbed vegetable or meat with a single-herb salad dressing. More spicy herbs can be used in dessert. It is not good to mix too many different herbs and seasonings — especially those with conflicting strong flavor in one dish. Dillweed and caraway, for example, seem to fight with one another. The general amounts of dry herbs versus fresh ones would be one part dry to three parts fresh — 1/8 teaspoon garlic powder equals a medium clove. It takes about ¼ teaspoon dry herb or spice per pound of meat or per medium sauce pan of vegetable except for pepper, cayenne and garlic, which require less, about 1/8 teaspoon. When adding herbs to cold salad dressings or foods, add them several hours before serving so that the flavor has a chance to be released and blended.

A tasty Italian seasoning for salad dressings could include basil, oregano, marjoram, chervil and garlic if desired. French dressing usually includes oregano, sage, basil, and rosemary. A salad dressing blend excellent for cottage cheese or yogurt is basil, tarragon, parsley, marjoram and rosemary. If you want a taste treat, try this blend cooked on vegetables — carrots or brocoli — and add some mushrooms and onions.

There are some excellent concentrated vegetable broth powders on the market, either in bulk or in name brands, which make an excellent salt substitute. Powdered kelp is also a good salt substitute. The less vegetables are cooked, the less salt they require as they have their own natural salt flavor. Celery salt, too, can be used as a substitute to cut down on salt. Celery seed comes from

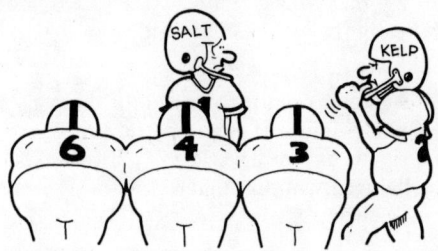

wild celery related to the parsley family, not from celery. The tiny seeds have a mildly sweet but intense flavor. If you want a new taste treat, add celery seed to your fruit salad. Celery salt is also good in potato salad and can be used with other herb mixtures in vegetable dishes in the same way that garlic is used.

Monosodium glutamate has been used for a long time to enhance the flavor of foods. It is actually a salt (sodium salt of glutamic acid, an amino acid). Sugar beets, wheat and corn are its major sources.

Interesting Facts About Condiment Herbs

Chili Powder can be made by blending chili peppers, ground cumin, oregano and garlic powder. Sometimes the addition of allspice, onions and cloves can be included.

Coriander leaves or Chinese parsley has a somewhat pungent, bitter taste and is a favorite herb used in Latin American, Chinese, Russian and East European dishes.

Cumin is the Spanish herb to give the taste of enchilada. Cumin does wonderful things to a tomato sauce, but can also be used alone in cooked vegetables, adding garlic also if one wishes. Cumin is especially delicious on cooked corn.

Curry is a flavor little used in America but is widely used in the Middle East, India, Europe, and the Orient. It gives a wonderful flavor when added to vegetable dishes. With strong flavors such as broccoli, cabbage or cauliflower, curry and mushroom makes an interesting new experience in flavor. Curry powder is a blend of from 16 to 20 pungent herbs and spices usually including coriander seed, cloves, black pepper, chilies, celery seed, cumin, cardamon, caraway seed, cinnamon, fennel seed, fenugreek seed, ginger, mace, mint leaves, mustard seed, nutmeg, poppy seed, saffron, sesame seed and leaves from the 'curry tree' (*Murraya koenigii*). Curry grows in tropical Hindustan, and at the foot of the Himalayas in India. It is a specialty in cocktail sauces or salad dressings.

Garlic, Black Pepper and *Cayenne* are the old stand-bys when it comes to flavoring meats, vegetables and salads, but when one learns to add other herbs to these, the difference will surprise and please one's family.

Marjoram, cousin to oregano, was used historically for religious purposes and as a medicine. It is interesting how most all condiments and aromatic herbs aid digestion — marjoram is one in particular and is excellent for sour stomach, loss of appetite or indigestion.

Oregano is the pizza herb and it will be fun for you to discover how one can enhance the flavor of vegetables by adding oregano and garlic either to a tomato sauce for sprinkling over or to add after cooking.

Parsley always makes a nice addition to vegetables or salads and is one of the richest known sources of Vitamin A. Too often we use it only for decoration and fail to receive the benefits from eating this decoration, both in taste and improved health.

Poppy seed comes from the poppy which produces opium. The seed, however, does not have the opium qualities, so there is no narcotic effect from eating the seed. They have been used for topping on baked goods, but here again is another very fine addition to a vegetable dish or salad. Many other seeds have become popular additions and toppings for salads and vegetable dishes such as chia seed, sunflower, pumpkin seeds, sesame and dillweed — each adding not only taste but nutritional value.

Rosemary is an old fashioned remedy for colds, headache and nervousness. It has been used as a mouth wash for bad breath and sore throat. It has even been used as a shampoo, been found to strengthen the eyes, and is helpful in cases of coughs or insanity. Rosemary, as with so many other condiment aromatic herbs, aids digestion.

Saffron is the most expensive spice herb and comes from a flower requiring 225,000 flowers to produce one pound of saffron. A little goes a long way in flavoring, but saffron aids in the digestion of oil and removes not only cholesterol but gallstones when taken in large amounts. When taken hot, it produces perspiration.

Savory is an herb of the mint family used in chowders, stuffings and baked beans. It creates a tasty treat when added to fresh lima beans or peas with marjoram, oregano and a little white onion.

Thyme is another herb useful as a condiment and a medicine; it is a reliable nervine, always a good remedy for gas, weak stomach and cramps of the stomach, and will relieve headaches. It is used often with tarragon. Some vegetables with which it blends well are asparagus, beets, green beans, and butternut squash.

Vegetables and their Compatible Herbs and Spices

Avocados: dillweed, basil, oregano, soup broth.

Beets: dillweed, mint, marjoram.

Brussel sprouts: sage, dillweed, marjoram, oregano.

Carrots: mint, thyme, dillweed, marjoram.

Cauliflower: basil, tarragon, rosemary, cumin, savory.

Celery: thyme, dillweed, mint.

Corn: marjoram, rosemary, dill.

Cucumbers: basil, oregano, mint.

Eggplant: oregano, basil, thyme, saffron.

Green beans: tarragon, basil, dillweed, dry mustard.

Lima beans: savory, marjoram, oregano.

Mayonnaise: bay leaves, oregano, mint, dillweed, dry mustard.

Okra: bay leaves, thyme, saffron.

Onions: basil, oregano, thyme.

Parsnips: marjoram, tarragon.

Peas:	oregano, chervil, savory, bay leaves, thyme, rosemary.
Peppers:	basil, oregano, thyme.
Potatoes (sweet):	honey, cinnamon, nutmeg, ginger, mint, marjoram.
Potatoes (white):	basil, dillweed, savory, tarragon.
Summer Squash:	sage, thyme.
Tomatoes:	basil, cumin, ginger, nutmeg, oregano, tarragon.
Winter squash:	honey and spices, allspice, anise, cinnamon, cloves, ginger, nutmeg or basil, chervil, mint, oregano, tarragon.
Yellow hookneck squash:	sage, thyme.
Apple cider: (warm)	place cinnamon sticks, whole cloves and whole nutmeg in a cloth bag to be added to cider as it is being warmed.
Fruit drinks:	allspice, cinnamon, ginger, nutmeg.
Green beans:	tarragon, basil, dillweed, thyme.
Potatoes (white):	basil, dillweed, savory, tarragon.
Fruit and fruit salad:	flavor is enhanced by honey rather than sugar as honey allows the fruit taste to remain while sugar causes the fruit taste to go flat.

Most cooked vegetables go well with tomato sauce, onions or garlic — along with the herbs.

There is something charming that fills the heart with gladness, when one surrounds his or her life with the fragrance of herbs and spices. It is like wearing a heavenly perfume. Experiment with herbs and you will become aware of this special feeling.

COSMETIC HERBS

Cosmetics are not new, but have been used for thousands of years. Records show that the ancient Egyptians applied cosmetics as early as 4,000 B.C. They were used for decoration, protection against the sun's rays, dry climate and for religious purposes. The Romans, Greeks and Egyptians made their cosmetics from herbs and plants, using powdered minerals to make hair dyes, eye makeup, face powder and paints. Early African and American Indian cultures painted their bodies in war time and for magical ceremonies.

The word "cosmetic" was created from the Greek word, "kosmos," which means "adornment" or "order." "Cosmetics" include face powder, face makeup, lipstick, rouge, nail polish, eye makeup, toothpaste, shampoo, perfume, skin creams, astringents, bath oils, hair removers, shaving cream, tanning lotion, hair sprays, oils, hair dyes, permanents and soap. There are more than 5,000 ingredients used by manufacturers in producing the many varieties and brands of body adornments and care.

Skin care products have always been sold based on the same premises that the drug companies have sold drugs — treat the effect, rather than the cause. Cosmetics work on the the superficial surface, rather than cleaning and healing the whole body and thereby making a more permanent change in the appearance of the skin. Cosmetics are not the answer to skin care problems.

There are many simple, less expensive natural ingredients that can be used on the skin better than the waxy substances used in many high priced products. Olive oil, for example, is one of the best oils for feeding and softening the skin. Massage therapists, who use mineral oils as a lubricant, will have cracking, rough, sore hands from constant use of mineral oils, while the therapist who uses olive oil has soft, smooth hands.

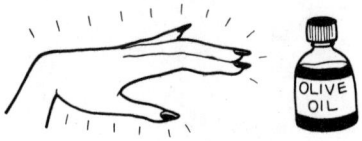

There are many other fine oils that can be used to feed, smooth, and protect the skin — such as soy oil, sesame seed, safflower and even pumpkin seed oil. Pumpkin seed oil will kill any parasites living under the skin and will clean skin that does not respond completely to an improved diet. Pumpkin seed oil can even stop a yeast infection, because of its ability to kill parasites. Chapparal also kills parasites under the skin, making it one of the best herbs for clearing skin.

A very effective skin bath for eczema and rashes of all kinds is equal parts of echinacea, golden seal, yellow dock, burdock root and witch hazel bark. Use a heaping tablespoon of the mixture to a pint of boiling water, remove from heat and steep for a half hour. Apply several times a day on affected parts.

During the teen years, acne can pit and scar the face for life and it has become a universal problem which helps the sale of skin creams and medications. Unfortunately, these medications do not solve the problem. Acne seems to have become more of a problem during the last 20 years, as young people are increasingly dependent on junk food. An acne sufferer can clean up his skin quickly when the diet is changed to fruits, vegetables, seeds and nuts.

When I was a child, my father was a sales manager for a large cosemtics company. He traveled all over training salesmen and groups of women how to care for their skin. While making a sales advertising film, he decided to show the skin of a child, so he used me in the film. It was at this time that he impressed upon me how to care for my skin. I remember well the pictures of women with blackheads, pimples, dry and oily skin. After seeing how bad the skin can become, I decided I would always follow his advice.

The first step he maintained was to clean the face thoroughly. The face should never be washed with warm water because warm water is often the cause of large pores. Soap the face with a good soap, then rinse thoroughly by cupping the hands and covering the face with cold water many times until it is what he called "squeaky clean." Always use a good astringent and a good moisture cream.

My father also said that it was important for a man to use only cold water to shave because it made the beard stand up. He had a heavy beard and always used cold water. He taught me that most men use an astringent on their beard, but do not put it on their face and nose; consequently you see so many men with large, unsightly pores. Facial skin care is just as necessary for a man as for a woman.

It was at this period in my life that he taught me to use a clay pack mask occasionally and to be selective about the cosmetics I purchased. Since I was a child I have always washed my face with cold water. Warm or hot water causes the skin to become saggy and soft, while cold water tones and tightens. People who take too many hot baths or showers cause their skin to become loose and wrinkled. Even up to the time of my father's death he did not have saggy, loose skin on his face or around his chin.

When certain herbs are added to the diet, such as chapparal (6 to 8 capsules a day), or an herbal pumpkin formula (mentioned below), the skin clears even more quickly.

It is always helpful to use an overall body cleanser to help clear the skin, such as the following:

Culver's root — 1 part
Mandrake — 1 part
Violet leaves — 1 part
Poke root — 1/8 part
Cascara sagrada — 1/8 part
Witch hazel bark — 1/8 part
Mullein — 1/8 part
Comfrey — 1/8 part
Slippery elm — 1/8 part

Take 6 capsules daily

One of the Vitamin B factors is paba (para amino benzoic acid). Eczema or a skin pigmentation disease, such as vitillige, can be helped by paba. Paba also prevents sunburn for fair skinned people.

Some herbs which will help to purify the blood (and in the process help to beautify and cleanse the skin), as well as to be used as a poultice, wash, or ointment follow:

Red clover — skin cancer, also relevant to nervous system
Buckthorn bark — general blood purifier
Burdock root — general blood purifier
Cleavers — general blood purifier
Dandelion — removes uric acid
Saffron — cleans the liver
Golden seal — antibiotic
Vervain — acts on the nervous system.
(Some skin diseases are caused from a fault in the nervous system.)
Oregon grape — general blood purifier
Poke root — kills parasites, itching, eczema
Plantain — wounds, burns, running sores, eczema, itching
Chickweed — used in small amounts, at first acts as an anti-allergic herb. Some skin diseases are caused because the body is toxic and the bowel and kidneys are not carrying off the waste and certain foods.
Hyssop — general blood purifier
Wintergreen — kills parasites
Elder flowers — itching skin

Bayberry — good for ringworm, gangrenous sores, boils, carbuncles and infections.

Some of the herbs that have been used successfully in treating skin diseases are:

Golden seal — Skin rash and running sores, wounds, or abrasions. Use the powdered herb directly on the skin. Golden seal has an antibiotic property which stops infections.

Cayenne — Stops bleeding of a wound. Apply directly on the wound.

Bittersweet — for eczema and ulcers

Borage — for ringworm, ulcers

Chamomile — for gangrenous sores and wounds

Celadine — eczema

Comfrey — burns, ulcers, gangrenous sores

Flaxseed — abscesses, boils

Mugwart — bruises, abscesses and boils

Sarsaparilla — ringworm

Sassafras — varicose ulcers

Slippery elm — boils

Herbs can also be used for hair care. Henna leaves color the hair red. Nettle and rosemary prevent hair from falling out when taken internally or when used as a rinse. Made into tea, sage, peach leaves, and burdock leaves are an excellent rinse and are useful when taken internally to beautify the hair. A tea made of the willow tree can cure dandruff. Marshmallow leaves made into a tea and used as a rinse will help to prevent hair from falling out. Many people today have dry, lifeless, colorless hair because of their poor internal condition. The deficiency of certain important vitamins and minerals can cause brittle, ugly hair lacking color and luster. Vitamins A, B2, B6, C and E (folic acid) are necessary for skin and hair beauty. Para-amino Benzoic acid or Paba is lacking when hair turns gray. Pantothenic acid is also called the antigraying vitamin.

Dandruff can be caused by the lack of magnesium in the body. Warts can be caused by the lack of Vitamin A. The lack of silicon causes boils on the skin.

The lack of sulphur causes the hair to be dull and lifeless. When adequate sulphur is used, the hair becomes glossy and beautiful. Sulphur is called the beautifying mineral. (A lack of sulphur is also responsible for unhealed sores.) Recent research has proven that zinc helps to beautify the hair.

Suntanning

We have been cautioned about skin cancer and too much sun. First of all, skin cancer is not caused by the sun, unless a person receives a severe burn. The sun is merely the drawing power which brings cancer already in the body to the surface. This is why a person who lives on a vegetable or fruit diet can take more exposure to the sun's rays. The heavy starch and meat eater would be more subject to skin cancer.

It used to be a necessary thing to work out in the sun. People covered their bodies and heads from exposure, but today suntanning is a popular sport. The skin will not become leathery or old-looking from tanning as long as water is used along with the sunning. A spray bottle of water or the hose can be used if no swimming pool, lake or beach is available. A good, soft oil such as sesame seed, corn, safflower, soy, or preferably olive oil can be used after the sun bath. Do not just put oil on and let the skin fry. Use water to maintain moisture, then apply the oil.

A clean, healthy body, made so from eating a good, nutritious diet filled with the vitamins and minerals of life food, is the real beginning to that beautiful color and transparent glow that goes with lovely skin. Real beauty literally comes from within.

NERVINE HERBS

The word disease means lack of ease. When we begin to be mentally disturbed, when we allow circumstances or people around us to disturb our minds and upset us, we lose inward peace. This is the beginning of disease and fear becomes the greatest of all diseases because it is the greatest disturber of the mind.

When we learn to have faith and a cheerful countenance to look for the positive, the happy, the good around us, the body begins to heal. The scriptures tell us: *"Whatsoever a man soweth, that shall he also reap."*

There is no escape from fundamental law. We cannot say, "I will just think myself into being able to put my finger in the electric socket and it will not hurt me."

Fear becomes the greatest of all diseases. Some people live out their entire lives in continual fear: Fear of the future, fear of poverty, fear of death, fear of what their friends or relatives may think, fear that they cannot keep up with the Joneses, afraid they will make a mistake in business or in many little daily tasks. People today are afraid of the poisons in their food, afraid of the contamination in the water and air, afraid of the danger of earthquakes, fire, flood, famine, war, and radioactive fallout. Most of all they fear germs and disease.

Fear is catching, and as these fearful ones send out their negative vibrations or express their fears, others quickly become charged with this most destructive of all forces. Fear becomes a universal, negative disease.

There are other laws of nature which must be obeyed. We cannot fill our bodies with filth or negative foods, chemicals and some of the rubbish that fills the shelves in the supermarkets. We cannot refuse to sleep or relax from work. We cannot refuse to exercise. We can become sick from the negative resulting from either the mental or the physical. Of the two, however, the mind is the more powerful.

We cannot experience joy in life when we fill our minds with hatred, strife, envy, and bitterness, selfishness or revenge. Peaceful tranquility comes only to those whose minds are filled with love, kindness, patience, tolerance and unselfishness. When Christ healed the sick, He said: *"Thy sins be forgiven thee."*

Disease is a sin. We may one day look upon sickness as sin when the world heals itself of all the filth and pain it now holds to itself. We may then find little sympathy for sickness. We may then ask what evil thoughts we have been thinking or what filthy thing have we been eating.

Thoughts are things as real as anything that can be seen with the eyes. Job said: *"Lo, the thing I greatly feared hath come upon me."* We attract to us that which we continually harbor, whether it is good or bad, positive or negative, and invariably we try to place the blame on circumstances or lady luck. Shakespeare said: *"Nothing is good or bad, but thinking makes it so."*

It would be useless to try to heal the nervous system without consideration of the mind. It would also be useless to heal the body without healing the nervous system.

The nerve force in the body must be strengthened if the body is to become well. To heal the nerve force in the body, be it mental, anxiety, anguish, fear, worry, or the nervous system itself, is the beginning of vital health. It is also the beginning of wisdom.

Because we are far from this high spiritual level, God placed all manner of herbs on the earth which would help us to relax, back up, calm down, and start over again. Some of the herbs which helped to give a new perspective, a calming, quieting effect, were called the nervine herbs. Each seem to have its own special way of acting upon the body or the mind. Some acted directly upon the physical body while others acted upon the emotions.

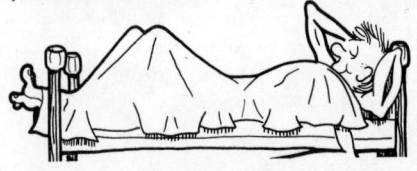

Catnip (Nepeta catoria). One of the oldest, most used home remedies. Used in tea or as an injection for the following:

Convulsions
Pain
Spasms
Gas
Acids in stomach caused from upset
Hysteria
Nervous headache
Colic
Inducing sleep

Chamomile (Anthemis nobilis). Has been used for centuries for babies and upset stomach.

Colic
Insomnia
Nervous indigestion
Neuralgia pain
(One of the old favorites as a home remedy)

Hops (Humulus lupulus). Has been used in a pillow to help insomnia. It can almost cause stupor and has been proven for many years. It is best taken in a tea form.

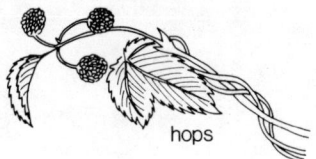
hops

Horsetail (Equisetum arvense). Often the thyroid can cause a nervous condition. Horsetail has a quieting effect on such a condition.
Nervous tension
Hysteria

Lobelia (Lobelia inflata). Large doses act as an emetic to empty the stomach, but a smaller dose acts on the nervous system in a most remarkable way, producing not only a profound state of relaxation but also seems to have the ability to move obstructions of waste matter, mucus, etc., from the body. For asthma and bronchial problems. Often insomnia is caused by upset stomach or congested liver and bowels. Lobelia has a way of cleaning as well as relaxing. The amount taken varies with each individual, but once a person finds the amount that is correct, it becomes a trusted friend. One of the best relaxants in the herb kingdom.

Mistletoe (Viscum album). Has been used and proven valuable for centuries as a remedy for nervous problems.

    Rheumatism
    Arthritis
    Mental upset
    Overactive brain

Nutmeg (Nux moschata). Has been used as a condiment or to aid digestion; is another fine sedative acting upon the nervous system calming:

    Stomach upset
    Gas
    Giddiness
    Stupor
    Delirium
    Indigestion
    Headache
    Bronchial asthma

Passion flower (Passiflora incarnta). Has been an antispasmodic and a powerful sedative.

    Produces rest
    Helps for nervous upset
    Hysteria
    Nervous asthma
    Insomnia
    Nervous excitement

Pulsatilla (Anemone pulsatilla).

    Crying
    Emotionalism
    Upset from pain
    Mental suffering from repentant grief

Rauwolfia (Rauwolfia serpentina). This wonderful herb has been known among herbalists for hundreds of years, but has recently made a new name in medicine because it was discovered by chemists to have a certain active ingredient which caused a pronounced tranquilizing effect. Because modern chemists take certain parts and isolate them to increase potency, this herb was of great interest to them. The isolated part was the alkaloid *(resperpine), (serpentinine)* or *(serpentine)*. These derivations are used extensively as a sedative considered of low toxicity.

Scullcap (Scutellaria lateriflora). One of the five tranquilizers.

Soothes the mind
Overcomes fear
Confusion
Headache caused from nervousness
Migraine headache

Valerian (Valerian officinalis). Seems to have an effect on the sensory nerves, so is useful for the following:

Pain
Twitching muscles
Gas
Dizziness
Hysteria
Upset
Light-headedness
Abdominal cramps
Spasms

Practice

DAD was a good doctor. Many times he sat by my bed and read or told me stories. I can still remember the touch of his hand on my forehead as he stroked my head until I fell asleep. I give thanks to God for such a father, who loved his children and taught them so many truths. Also, our diet was carefully planned by my knowledgeable mother to include the necessary nutritional foods. Our diet consisted of a bowl of whole wheat mush and a glass of alfalfa mint tea and honey for breakfast; home-made whole wheat bread, lots of fruits and vegetables, herb tea and milk, meat only on Sunday and never in the summer, and cakes or cookies made of whole wheat and honey. Still, I was often sick with earaches, broken ear drum, near mastoid and swollen glands — I suppose I was the weakest of the five children. It was not until I realized I was not strong enough to handle meat, milk and bread that I began to have good health.

Remembering back to my childhood, I recall my father saying so many times, **"The majority are always wrong." I feel inclined to** agree with his philosophy. When it comes to the important decisions, the majority seem to have an uncanny way of making the wrong choices. When the decisions are made incorrectly, the majority seem to be already conditioned to failure or at least to being mildly unhappy. When there are big, personal, world shaking choices to make, the majority have not been well enough informed to make such decisions to their advantage. In this world there are those few who are "seekers after truth," a special breed of individuals who have the courage of their convictions.

Often as we live from day-to-day, we reach a point in our lives where a choice is forced upon us and we are faced with two fateful alternatives. When the doctor announces that we must have a serious operation before we can continue, it is a frightening thing and a difficult decision to make.

Over the past 50 years people have become so dependent on what is considered good medical care, that unless one is an adventurous and truth seeking type of person, he would rarely consider trying an herbal formula or a natural method to help himself. When the rewards are so great and the outcome so much like a miracle, it is hard to understand why so few people have had the courage to try such methods.

Dr. Samuel Thompson's life was filled with many hardships, both as a child and as an adult. Because of an analytical, scientific mind, coupled with the same spirituality I have observed in the other physicians of the past, he seemed quickly and easily to draw a correct conclusion. He could see how by natural herbal methods and correct laws, marvelous results could be achieved. It is difficult to imagine how the doctors of his day could maintain their integrity with such pretensions as they made dabbling in the art of healing. Despite heavy pressures from the growing established medical practices of his time, he continued to help whenever he could, always confident that his best tool was truth. He was an uneducated man as to accredited schooling. His education had been practical from a childhood knowledge of the use and handling of herbs on into his adult practice of helping and serving the sick. He seemed to be compelled by the knowledge he possessed to continue to serve mankind regardless of the consequences to himself. His aim was apparently worthy of the sacrifice of his individual advantage.

As I read the narrative of his own life, I see such a parallel today with the many naturopathics who have been so persecuted for their knowledge of the truth. Such a lonely ordeal they have faced because they have touched the most sensitive nerve which today causes us to be trapped into chemical therapy (big money). Understanding how the body feeds and eliminates would cause us to recognize that elimination is not a side effect at all, but rather nature's way to rid us of those elements causing pain or obstruction in the body. Some herbs are more laxative than others, so if it were understood to let nature, along with herbs, slowly remove obstruction, we would all have the good sense not to take too much that is highly laxative and move waste faster than the body's ability to rebuild or throw it out.

Willard Richards and Priddy Meeks were a part of the first medical society in Utah. Both were herbalists. Willard Richards also had the training of a medical doctor to use the drugs of his day, but he believed only in the use of mild herbal medicines. He learned about lobelia from Dr. Samuel Thompson and regarded it highly. Willard Richards had seen his sister go down hill physically with cancer of the breast using the new drug medicine of the day until the doctor finally decided to remove the breast. Willard had loved this older sister as a mother and was asked to stand in to help hold her down while the breast was removed without any anesthetic. This experience was sheer torture to his soul and he felt that certainly God could provide a better way than that to cure cancer. One day when he was traveling from town-to-town giving lectures and demonstrating the marvels of electricity, he arrived at a small town and came upon a mob of men dragging a poor man to jail. Upon inquiring as to why the man was being so badly treated, he was told that this was Dr. Thompson, a quack who said he could heal cancer with lobelia. Being a curious and learned man, he was immediately intrigued by the prospect of a cure for cancer.

When Dr. Thompson was incarcerated, one of his first visitors was Willard Richards. After being satisfied that the method worked, he asked for permission to use the method which was in those days always protected under government patent. The method was called the Thompsonian medicine and was used in the early pioneer days in the Salt Lake Valley.

Modern-day Example

It may be interesting to read a personal story about the removal of gallstones through a simple, natural method. This lady said the entire procedure cost her a total of $14.00 and only a few days of time as compared to the pain, suffering and expense of surgery.

> "January 1, 1975, was the beginning of a new life for me. I weighed well in excess of 250 lbs. and needed an operation for gallstones; however there had to be an easier way — there were too many obstacles standing in the way. To mention but a few: overweight, chemical imbalance in my body, reaction to drugs, recovery time, loss of income during recovery, needed baby sitters and most important to myself was the fear of the operation. I was not willing to undergo what seemed, to me, a senseless battle. I didn't mind the stones being removed, but I was not willing to part with my gallbladder. It was mine and I wanted the continued function that it served within my body.
>
> Just a few days before the year 1975 was closing its books of time — to rally in the new year, I drove (not trotted) to a local health food store and asked advice. Then as the old year was bidding its good-byes, I too was bidding my good-byes to some old habits and much needed change. Change in views, mind and diet.
>
> The following then is a copy of the information I

gathered that day from the health food store. The first three (3) days alternate every hour, 8 oz. of apple concentrate, diluted according to directions, with water, distilled if possible. On third night, drink four oz. cold pressed olive oil mixed thoroughly with four oz. of fresh grapefruit juice. Gallstones will be eliminated next day... they float, look waxy, various shades of green.

On fourth day for breakfast eat raw fruit, for lunch fruit and for dinner, fruit. On the fifth day for breakfast eat raw fruit, lunch, salad, and for dinner, fruit. On the sixth day for breakfast eat raw fruit, for lunch a salad and for dinner, fruit salad or slightly steamed vegetables. Fruit and salad ingredients are raw; only two or three at a time. Do not use bananas, head lettuce, or potatoes (unless raw). Dressing, just cold pressed oil and lemon juice.

Every night use herb laxative, enema, douche, sitz bath. Sitz bath — sideways in the tub, legs out, sit in warm water 10-15 minutes and then quickly in cold for three — four minutes. Douche — Warm water or yellow dock tea or teaspoon apple cider vinegar in one quart water. Enema — warm water.

On December 31, 1975, being my third night, I drank the ½ cup cold pressed oil and ½ cup fresh grapefruit juice. This was the biggest pain I went through. It took two hours of courage and much inspiration. How could anything so simple work so well? Around 4 p.m. in the afternoon, New Years Day, I passed stones in various sizes — ranging from that of a large red grape, sizes of seedless grapes, raisin size and that of smaller sizes resembling tiny peas in a pod and smaller. Over 80 stones were passed in that one elimination. Later in the evening brought another elimination and well over 50 stones, again in various sizes. At this point, I felt from within there were more stones, and for this reason altered the course of the above information obtained from the health food store. That evening again I drank ½ cup cold pressed olive oil and this time ½ cup lemon juice. The next day there were over 50 stones passed in the elimination. That night ½ cup pressed olive oil and this time ½ cup fresh grapefruit juice. The results the next day were some 20 odd stones of various size. That night I took ½ cup of fresh lemon juice. Next day's elimination consisted of one stone. I now felt, from within, that all stones were going to come out.

A short time later for my own peace of mind, in being absolutely sure, I did have an X-ray and found two stones remaining of somewhat larger size. Fresh apple juice has helped in softening these larger stones and I have had no trouble with my gallbladder since. I have since carried a child full term and had absolutely no problem with the gallbladder whatsoever. This is a testmony to me, for I had been told I couldn't carry a child until the gallbladder* was removed."

When such a simple method for removal of gallstones is made known, it is still a frightening prospect to the majority. There are, however, more and more people taking courage from these people who give testimonies of their experiences.

Van Wyck Brooks wrote:

"How delightful is the company of generous people who overlook trifles and keep their minds instinctively fixed on whatever is good and positive in the world about them. People of small calibre are always carping. They are bent on showing their own superiority, their knowledge or prowess or good breeding. But magnanimous people have no vanity, they have no jealousy, they have no reserves, and they feed on the true and the solid wherever they find it. And, what is more, they find it everywhere."

SPECIAL NOTE
*The gallbladder is part of the bilinary system, whose concern is drawing bile from the liver, storing and concentrating it and ultimately conveying it to the intestines. Bile is brought into the duodenum from the gallbladder, because of oil in the diet, in order to digest and properly use oils. The bile is collected in the liver by small ducts. There they coalesce forming 2 large ducts. The liver then appears to have a deep fissure called the porta hepatis. The portal artery with accompanying nerve plexures, veins and small lymphatic vessels are admitted at this place on the liver. Right and left hepatic ducts after they leave the porta hepatis, unite to form the common hepatic duct. There is a continuous flow of bile in this duct down to the duodenum. The cystic duct leading from the gallbladder runs into the common duct which runs into the pancreas before the duct empties at the duodenum. The gallbladder is a sac, with only one way out through the cystic duct. The gallbladder's function is to discharge stored bile at necessary intervals. The gallbladder's complete constriction (emptying) is caused by heavy oil foods, meat, fat and egg yolks. The liver will then send more bile trickling down the common hepatic duct. This does not allow it to escape into the duodenum because of a msucle called the *bilany sphincter* which closes the bile duct causing the bile to find its way up the cystic duct into the gallbladder. The signal is given before a meal from the brain, via the vagus nerve from the intestines, to call upon a hormone called *cholecystokynin* to activate

the process. Large amounts of oil cause the gallbladder to flush. Oil is repellent to the gallbladder. You might say similarly, the way water is repellent to the colon — causing it to empty quickly. When the gallbladder is removed, the normal liver functions are confused.

The herb saffron is also helpful in overcoming gallstones, as it works on the liver, somehow correcting its function. The cause of gallstones is too much starch and meat in the diet. The use of lemon or grapefruit, used with the oil, merely acts as an alkalizer so that so much oil will not cause nausea.

Work and Growth

If we want to accomplish things
we must ever be aware
That work and growth are synonomous.
They make a mighty pair.

Conclusion

RECENTLY as I was walking out of a grocery store, a sharp, almost angry voice behind me said, "Can I get through?" As I opened the door for her, my heart went out to this haggard, upset mother juggling a large sack of groceries in one arm and a wallet and soda pop in the other. Behind her screaming in a tantrum of pain with tears streaming down his face was her two-or three-year-old son hugging a soda pop to his breast and demanding the money to buy penny gum. In her desperation the mother awkwardly shifted her load so as to take some pennies from her purse. The boy snatched the pennies and stopped crying, going quickly back into the store leaving his mother with a drained look of relief. When I am asked to speak on local television and radio stations as I travel across the country, I feel like making a special plea to somehow save the children. The fact that children have arthritis and cancer becomes a frightening question as to how the following generations are going to survive the birth defects and physical problems of such a weak people.

Our hospitals are full to overflowing, our institutions for brain-damaged retarded children have cropped up everywhere like mushrooms. We have spent millions and gathered millions to try to rehabilitate children with whom even their own families cannot cope. Our fund raising organizations gather millions for so called research to find answers to cancer, arthritis, muscular dystrophy, leukemia, and diabetes. We are a charitable nation, and we keep contributing to every cause in the hope that someone will find the answer. Our health problems of the past fifty years of drug use and abuse have only compounded. All of the major "old people" diseases have become children's diseases.

Sundays in church afford me the greatest opportunity to observe children in company with their parents. I have observed over the past few years that as the children become sicker or more hyperactive, their parents seem to pay less and less attention to their cries. Often the cry will reach a terrifying crescendo before mother or father finally takes little Johnny out, as if they were so accustomed to such weeping that they had turned him off. If it were only one or two children crying, a tolerant audience could be patient, but as the meeting progresses, the sound from every corner of the chapel becomes a wailing cry until it is with great difficulty that the speaker gets any attention at all.

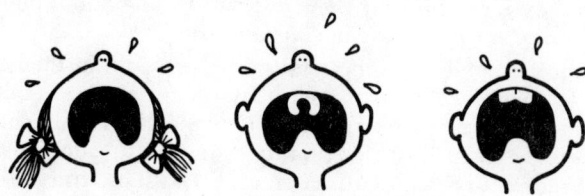

Once my son facetiously said, "These kids need a little helmet with an air bubble on the front where they are the only ones who can hear themselves." And I said, "Yeah, and with an ear plug to their parent's ear." Mother and Dad must be tuned out for sanity's sake. Has discipline turned to resignation when it is easier to turn them off than to endure the continual howling? Has it become easier to be like one of the latest television ads and give little son or daughter a piece of candy than to teach him to know that there are places in this world to be quiet and peaceful? Even though I see it all the time, I never cease to be shocked when a young mother with a hyperactive child, who can no longer be controlled, gives him a handful of candy to keep him quiet.

One young mother said to me recently, "I've got to go to work. I can't stand my kids. All they do is scream from morning to night." When she asked my advice I affectionately told her, "If you don't discipline them now, you will be running away from them the rest of their lives." On one of my trips home by plane from Chicago recently, I recall a mother and father wrestling a young screaming child most of the trip until everyone on the plane was upset. Finally in desperation the mother took a bottle of medicine from her purse and forced a spoonful down the child's throat. The child dropped off to sleep with such suddenness, he almost appeared to have fainted.

According to a Washington AP notice in a Salt Lake paper of October 28, 1977, the federal government is drafting consumer leaflets warning that tranquilizer users may become dependent on the drugs. Such drugs as Valium, Librium, and Meprobomate accounted for more than 520 million dollars in sales last year. The FDA said tranquilizers are the nation's most prescribed drugs.

Has discipline become impossible today because children are so irritable and half sick that their parents can no longer enjoy being parents? As I watch haggard, harrassed mothers and fathers in church try to give their children correct spiritual values, I wonder just how impressed these tantrum-oriented children really are in being exposed to what should be a spiritual atmosphere. It is pretty hard to talk about perfume and flowers to a man with a bad cold. To a person who has a volcano going on inside, love, peace and harmony mean nothing. It is difficult to talk about buoyant, abundant health to someone in constant pain.

As I look around at youngsters today I see pain in their faces, sadness in their eyes, despair and many other negative manifestations that should never be a part of a child's life. Happy children grow up to be happy, interested, interesting, useful adults. Are we raising children to be contentious and filled with bitterness as they become fully grown? Are the sins of this drug, junk-food generation of parents going to be visited upon the third and fourth generations until they make a reverse in this awful trend? It is my opinion that it is just as important to teach a child how to live physically as it is to teach him how to live spiritually. If parents are going to allow this vicious circle to continue by turning a deaf ear to the cries of their children and then blow all resolve of discipline by rewarding the tantrum with junk food or candy, what kind of people will we be living with in a few years?

Will the hyperactive drug addict ever know the sweetness of service, the quiet of solitude, the tenderness of harmonious love and the self-respect of a disciplined life? Will the brain-dysfunctioned person who lives on drugs ever know the joy of self-learning and self-disciplined accomplishment? Who are we kidding today when we take little Johnny to the doctor and say, "Give him something. I can't stand him"? Who is the teacher who really loves children who would say, "Take your child to the doctor. He needs drugs so I can cope with him." Where will all of today's child-addicts of five and six going to be at sixteen or seventeen? Undisciplined except with the drugs? Who are these people in the world of medicine or on the school boards of today who claim to be interested in the welfare of children, who perpetrate such an insidious plot against them? Drugs have become the modern methods to treat the new illness of either hyperactive or brain-dysfunctioned people.

We are not solving the problems, because we treat the effect rather than the cause. Therefore, we find the numbers increasing by leaps and bounds. Are we going to be able to treat all of our children with drugs? Do we really want that to be the answer? When I look back on the time I was raising my babies and being a full time mother, I reflect on that time as the happiest of my life. I love every minute of it. It is with sorrow that I wonder how many young mothers today are really enjoying the great privilege of motherhood. There were advantages of special knowledge that I had, however, that made my children well and happy, which I would like to share in this writing.

First of all, young mothers today have had to live through the penicillin age when they killed the germs but never cleaned out the problem. Disease has been looked upon as some kind of abstract demon waiting to pounce on some unsuspecting victim, and only the doctor had power over life and death with his war against

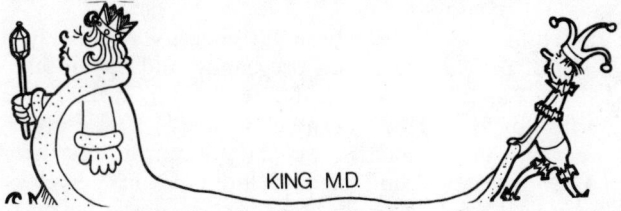

KING M.D.

germs. Never, until recently, has today's mother even supposed that what a person ate had anything whatsoever to do with health or sickness, so long as her child got enough protein-building blocks. She has been taught that a well-balanced diet was all that was necessary, with lots of protein. What is a well-balanced diet? Protein, carbohydrates, starch, vegetables. The best protein has been considered to be meat (no matter how many chemicals have been used to raise it) or milk. Carbohydrates mean anything sweet — fruit, sugar, cake, pie, cookies, candy, soda pop, honey, etc. Some vegetables were considered necessary and some starch — grains, cereals, bread, hot dog buns — all lumped into one part of a well-balanced diet. So if I ate a hot dog, soda pop and a salad with a candy bar for dessert, I was eating a well-balanced diet according to this absurd logic. Could this be why we have so many sick children? Isn't it time that we began to divide foods into better categories and find out how to obtain optimum health for our children?

In raising our six children we used doctors only to set a bone or sew an injury. The reason we didn't need them is that we fed them differently. We knew how to treat them when they got sick. *First* of all, a mother must understand how the body feeds and eliminates. (Refer to book *Is Any Sick Among You?*) She must understand that certain foods are more mucus-forming than others, thus making more food for germs and parasites. *Secondly*, she must know that in order to have good fuel for the body, food must be high in vitamin and mineral content and be able to be eliminated quickly from the body. Such foods have a built-in roughage which sweeps the colon clean like a broom. *Thirdly,* she must know the importance of live, raw food, which acts like a catalyst to move vitamins and minerals rapidly to the body cells.

A child should not have meat before the age of eight. Some pediatricians are learning that babies should not be glued up so they will sleep all night with a bowl of mush before bedtime. In fact they have discovered that a baby's digestive system cannot handle such concentrated starch at all. This is the cause of so many colds, bronchitis and pneumonia. I raised my babies on milk (breast milk) and raw blended fruit until they were a year old. After weaning them, I put one on carrot juice rather than milk, and the others on raw goat milk.

If the child tends to have bronchitis because of a sickly chronic condition of the mother during pregnancy, and the mother wishes to use carrot juice, a spoonful of soft, raw oil must be added to a daily intake of food. This oil can be blended in fresh fruit.

Science has pre-decided it was the protein in milk that babies needed. So when the child cannot handle the heavy hydrogenated pasteurized oils of cow's milk and seems to do better on the soft olive oils of a powdered formula, they assume they have solved the problem. It is not the protein, however, as much as it is the minerals, vitamins and oils that the baby needs. There we have been raising a lot of babies on skim milk or on a high protein diet lacking the live enzymes, minerals and vitamins of raw milk. In either case, we are raising mucus-filled or flabby, weak children subject to all manner of diseases. When the body is kept clean by foods that do not cause mucus and have sufficient mineral, vitamins and fatty acid oil content, a mother need no longer fear the microbe. Germs and parasites do not live on sound, healthy tissue. They live on the refuse-waste of the body.

My children did not have the childhood diseases the other children did, and they did not have to have immunizations. When my children were a year old, only vegetables were added to the diet of milk and fruit. Some were cooked and some were eaten raw. Soft oil was used on cooked vegetables. Milk was discontinued at three years old. Up to the age of three babies have an enzyme — gastric lipase — which digests fat in the stomach. After three, the liver bile digests the fat.

When milk products are placed in the sick adult body, they only add mucus. The protein requirements for man are definitely proven by the changes occurring in mother's milk at different stages in the development of the child. The amount of protein in mother's milk diminishes as the child grows older, starting with 2.38 per cent protein at birth and diminishing to 1.07 percent protein by six months of age. (Cow's milk is 16 percent protein.)

Children have a cold because the body has accumulated toxic waste, and the waste is being eliminated. If young mothers understood this one principle they would not be in such a hurry to feed their children on mucus-forming junk foods. Drugs, poisons on foods, commercial fertilizers, nutrition-poor foods, too many cooked, dead foods contribute to an accumulation of toxic waste in the body.

We can't always direct our children's diets because in-laws, teachers and well-meaning friends often feed them something wrong. Along with the commercial, nutritionally poor foods we have to buy at today's market (not to mention the residue of poison on foods) there is no way today to have immaculate health. So if we feed our children as has been explained, there should be no more than an occasional cold.

The Way to Treat a Cold

Using first of all an herbal laxative tea, for babies 1 oz. only which can be put into a bottle of alfalfa mint tea to overcome strong flavor with the addition of honey to sweeten. Then an hour later an enema, using small syringe. Test in book *Is Any Sick Among You?*, Page 147. 1,000 Vitamin C (not the coal tar product) to 2,000 milligrams an hour, and stop all milk or intake of solid food with the exception of fruit. Alfalfa mint tea and honey or juice may be used in baby's bottle. A cold can be overcome within a day or so by this method. Because we are unable to get proper organic foods, it is essential to add vitamins and minerals of a natural source to a child's diet on a regular basis. With older children who can take a capsule, golden seal is the best antibiotic for killing infection and germs. (Three capsules a day during a cold. I refer you to the section on vitamin deficiencies in my book *Is Any Sick Among You?*, Chapter 4.)

You may think that a fruit and milk diet, or fruit, vegetable, and milk diet would be lacking in Vitamin B. It has been established and proven that there is more Vitamin B in an apple than in a slice of bread. When children get plenty of fruit, their sweet tooth will be satisfied and the nervous system will be strengthened.

The tragedy of our times is that we are expecting that by 1980 one out of five Americans will have diabetes. It will not only be diabetes, but hyperactive children and adults because of the high sugar content in today's daily diet. Too much sugar leaches Vitamin B and calcium out of the body, leaving the nerves sick and the child hyperactive. Then we compound the problem by giving the child drugs which destroy Vitamins B and E. As I look upon the accepted care and nutrition for children I feel it borders on insanity.

A child who is hyperactive is a sick child in need of nourishment, particularly the B vitamins and calcium.

The following serve as natural tranquilizers for hyperactivity: Vitamin B Complex and calcium lactate or calcium gluconate taken over and above a daily multiple vitamin. Depending upon how nervous the child is, two to six tablets of each daily or as needed, two of each at a time. For babies and small children there are many good natural rice bran syrups or B-Complex syrups. A teaspoon is usually equal to two tablets. There are also calciums in powder form which can be added to fruit blends or juice. Carrot juice is one of the richest sources of natural calcium. Vitamin B complex and calcium is the best tranquilizer to be found.

Some herbs that feed and relax the nervous system for the hyperactive are red clover, catnip, lobelia, valerian, chamomile, lady slipper, mistletoe, hops, wood betony, and scullcap. These are all active nervine herbs. They can be used in formula or separately, up to six capsules a day. For babies, teas can be used (steeped, never boiled). Hops, catnip, chamomile or red clover are the best, as they are sweeter tasting and baby will take them better. Use a little honey to sweeten. Honey will not act in such a way as to leach Vitamin B the way sugar does.

Where there has been any brain damage, lady slipper acts the best. One to four capsules a day taken throughout the day. There is no danger in taking more if needed. With the combination of B, calcium, and herbs, it is usually unnecessary to take more. The brain-dysfunctioned child will particularly respond to a fruit and vegetable diet and will think more clearly and be more alert. With the addition of vitamins and minerals, lots of raw vegetable juice and two or three capsules of cayenne daily. He will be much improved.

Medical Science's idea for brain-dysfunction is to give speed (drugs). What a terrible thing to do to anyone, especially a defenseless child! Where else do helpless babies and children have to turn but to their parents when a tornado is going on inside of them? Do we contribute to it by what we feed them? Do we ignore the problems and let the children go undisciplined? Do we turn off their cry? Do we love them? If we do, it is time we learned to help, not hinder them.

If I were a young mother raising my family today without the knowledge I have had, it would be a most frightening prospect. Let's make changes for the better. Let's save the children.

It is worth the risk to learn to do some things for ourselves so as not to lean so heavily upon someone else to save our bodies. It is worth the sacrifice of junk food to be free of aches and pains. It is worth trying to use herbs because there is no danger of side effects — mistakes are not fatal. Finally it is worth knowing how to care for one's own body even if from purely economic standpoint.

Where There's a Will

The will to do is what it takes,
Don't quit 'cause you make mistakes
They can be a boon to you,
If you'll keep the will to do.

RECOMMENDED READING

Airola, Paavo. HOW TO GET WELL. Phoenix: Health Plus, 1975.

Ehret, Arnold. MUCUSLESS-DIET HEALING SYSTEM. Beaumont, Cal.: Ehret, 1953.

Griffin, LaDean. EYES: WINDOWS OF THE BODY AND THE SOUL. Provo: Bi-World, 1976.

Griffin, LaDean. IS ANY SICK AMONG YOU? Provo, Utah: Bi-World, 1974.

Griffin, LaDean. NO SIDE EFFECTS: THE RETURN TO HERBAL MEDICINE. Provo, Utah: Bi-World, 1975.

THE HERBALIST MAGAZINE. Provo: Bi-World, 1976–.

Illich, Ivan. MEDICAL NEMESIS. New York: Bantam Books, 1977.

Kloss, Jethro. BACK TO EDEN. Coalmont, Tenn.: Longview, 1969.

PREVENTION: THE MAGAZINE FOR BETTER HEALTH. Emmaus, PA.

INDEX

ABSCESSES 64
ACIDOSIS 67
ACNE 20, 39, 62
ACTH 27
ADDISON'S DISEASE 43
ADRENAL MALFUNCTION 42, 52
ALFALFA 20, 21, 25, 28
ALFALFA SPROUTS 27
ALLERGY 63
ALLSPICE 60
ANISE 60
ANTIBIOTIC HERB 36, 63, 64
ANTISPASMODIC HERB 29, 68
APPETITE 58
APPLE CIDER 60
AROMATIC HERBS 57
ARTERIOSCLEROSIS 5
ARTHRITIS 26, 53, 68
ASPEN 24
ASTHMA 33, 47, 67, 68
AVOCADOS 59

BABIES 67
BACTERIA 23
BAD BREATH 58
BARBITURIC ACID 9
BASIL 59, 60
BAY LEAVES 59, 60
BAYBERRY 64
BEARSFOOT 24
BEAUTY 3
BED WETTING 20
BEETS 59
BELLADONNA 9
BENSON, EZRA TAFT 34
BIO-RHYTHMS 2
BITTERSWEET 64
BLACK COHOSH 29
BLACK PEPPER 58
BLACK WALNUT 21, 24, 42
BLADDER 31
BLADDER RETENTION 20

BLADDERWRACK 19, 20
BLEEDING 64
BLOOD PURIFIERS 63
BLOOD SUGAR CONTROL 33
BLUE FLAG 24
BODY, A TEMPLE 1
BOILS 64
BORAGE 64
BRAIN OVERACTIVITY 68
BRONCHITIS 67
BROOKS, VAN WYCK 74
BRUISES 64
BRUSSEL SPROUTS 59
BUCKTHORN BARK 63
BURDOCK ROOT 21, 63
BURNS 63, 64

CAFFEINE 10
CALCIUM 21
CARBUNCLES 64
CARROTS 59
CATNIP 51, 67, 82
CAULIFLOWER 59
CAYENNE 19, 47, 58, 64
CEDAR BERRIES 36
CELADINE 64
CELERY 57, 59
CHAMOMILE 21, 64, 67, 82
CHAPPARAL 24, 62
CHERVIL 60
CHIA SEEDS 58
CHICKWEED 21, 63
CHILDHOOD DISEASE 70, 76
CHILI POWDER 57
CHINA, AND GINSENG 32
CHLORAL HYDRATE 10
CHLORAMPHENICOL 5
CHOLERA 23
CHOLESTEROL 59
CHOROID PLEXES GLAND 7
CINNAMON 60
CLEANSING 24
CLEAVERS 63

CLOVES 60
COLDS 26, 58, 81
COLIC 26, 27
COLON, TOXIC 3
COMFREY 64
CONDIMENT HERBS 56
CONFUSION 69
CONSUMPTION 33
CONVULSIONS 29, 67
COOKING, WITH CONDIMENTS 56
CORIANDER LEAVES 57
CORN 59
CORTISONE 43
COSMETIC HERBS 61
COUGHS 58
CRAMPS 20, 30, 69
CRETINISM 40
CRIME, AND USE OF SUGAR 34
CRYING 68
CUCUMBERS 59
CUMIN 57, 59, 60
CURRY 57
CUSHING'S DISEASE 26
CYCLE OF LIFE 2
CYSTIC FIBROSIS 5

DANDELION 19, 21, 22, 52, 63
DANDRUFF 64
DELIRIUM 68
DEMULCENT HERB 42
DERMATITIS WRINKLES 20
DIABETES 33, 81
DIAPHORETIC HERB 29
DIET 1; AND CHILDREN 79
DIGESTION 32, 50, 54, 58, 68
DILLWEED 58, 59, 60
DISEASE, AND FEAR 65
DIURETIC HERB 37
DIZZINESS 69
DRUG WITHDRAWAL 47
DRUGS, AND CHILDREN 77; VERSUS HERBS 13; SIDE EFFECTS, 9ff; TREATMENT OF CYSTIC FIBROSIS, 5

DULSE 19, 20, 21, 24, 38

ECZEMA 39, 62, 63, 64; INFANT 20
EGGPLANT 59
ELDER 20, 63
EMETIC HERB 67
EMOTIONS 66, 68
EMPHYSEMA 47
ERYTHROMYCIN 5
ESTROGEN, AND BLACK COHOSH 29
EXOCRINE GLANDS 5
EYEBRIGHT 19
EYES 38, 39
FACIAL OILINESS 20
FAINTING 20
FAITH 3
FEAR 69
FEAR, AND DISEASE 65
FEMALE PROBLEMS 29
FENUGREEK 19
FEVERS 33
FLAXSEED 64
FRUIT DRINKS 60
FRUIT SALAD 60
GALL BLADDER 74
GALLSTONES 59, 72
GANGRENOUS SORES 64
GARLIC 25, 58
GAS 59, 67, 68, 69
GIDDINESS 68
GINGER 30, 60
GINSENG 30
GLANDULAR BALANCE 38
GLUCOSE 36
GOITER 38, 41
GOLDEN SEAL 33, 39, 63, 64
GONORRHEA 37
GOUT 51
GRAPE LEAVES 19
GREEN BEANS 59, 60
GRIEF 68

HAIR LOSS 20
HARROW 22
HEADACHE 58, 59, 68, 69
HERBAL PUMPKIN FORMULA 63
HERBS, DESCRIPTION 14 ff; ON VEGETABLES 59; VERSUS DRUGS 13
HEROIN ADDICTION 39
HONEY 60, 82
HOPS 67, 82
HORMONE BALANCE 27, 29ff
HORSETAIL 67
HYPERACTIVITY 76, 81
HYPERCALCEMIA 25
HYPERGLYCEMIA 38
HYPERINSULINISM 38
HYPOGLYCEMIA 20, 42
HYPOTHYROIDISM 40
HYSSOP 63
HYSTERIA 67, 68, 69
INDIGESTION 68
INFECTIONS 64
INSANITY 58
INSOMNIA 67, 68
INSULIN 33, 35
INTESTINAL BACTERIA 54
IODINE 21, 23, 38, 40
IRON 21
ITCHING 63
JAUNDICE 51
JUNIPER BERRIES 36
KELP 19, 20, 21, 24, 38, 40
KIDNEY STONES 53
KIDNEYS 31, 36, 51
KLOSS, JETHRO 48ff

LACTIC-ACID BUILDUP 52
LADY SLIPPER 8, 82
LAMBS QUARTER 19
LAXATIVE HERB 31
LEMON JUICE 73
LETTUCE 20, 21
LEUCORRHEA 37
LICORICE 21, 39, 44
LIMA BEANS 59
LIGHT-HEADEDNESS 69
LIVER 63
LOBELIA 47, 67, 82

MAGNESIUM 21
MANDRAKE 24
MARJORAM 58, 59, 60
"MASTERPIECES" (POEM) 6
MAYONNAISE 59
MEASLES 51
MEDICAL RESEARCH 51
MEDICINE, HERBS AND DRUGS 14ff
MEEKS, PRIDDY 47, 71
MENSTRUATION 29
MENTAL SUFFERING 68, 69
MIGRAINE HEADACHES 69
MILK 26
MINERALS 21ff
MINT 59, 60
MISTLETOE 22, 68, 82
MOCCASIN FLOWER 8
MONOSODIUM GLUTAMATE 57
MORPHINE 10
MOUTH SORE 20
MOUTHWASH 58
MUCUS MEMBRANE 38
MUGWART 64
MULLEIN 21
MUSCLE CRAMPS 20
MUSCLE SPASMS 27
MUSTARD 59
MYXEDEMA 40
MYRRH 39

NARCOTIC ALKALOID 7
NERVOUS DISORDERS 20, 47, 58, 63, 66, 68, 82
NERVOUS HEADACHE 67, 69
NERVOUS INDIGESTION 67
NERVINE HERBS 59, 65
NETTLE 21
NEURALGIA 67
NEURITIS 20
NUTMEG 60, 68

OILS 61
OKRA 19, 59
OLIVE OIL 73
ONIONS 59
OREGANO 58, 59, 60
OREGON GRAPE 63
OSTEOPOROSIS 25
OXYTETRACYCLINE 6

PABA 63
PAIN 67, 68, 69
PARASITES 22, 63
PANCREAS 33
PAPRIKA 19
PARATHYROID 27
PARASITES 63; in diabetes 33
PARSLEY 19, 21, 22, 58
PARSNIPS 59
PASSION FLOWER 68
PEAS 60
PENTOBARBITAL 11
PEPPERS 60
PHENOBARBITAL 11
PHOSPHORUS 21
PINKHAM, LYDIA 29
PITUITARY GLAND 26
PLANTAIN 21, 22, 63
POKE ROOT 63
POPPY SEED 58
POTASSIUM 22, 31
POTATOES 60
PREGNANCY TOXEMIA 20
PROSTATE GLAND 30
PSORIASIS 20
PULSATILLA 68
PUMPKIN SEED 24, 31, 58
PYORRHEA 39
RASHES 62
RAUWOLFIA 68
RED CLOVER 63, 82
RED RASPBERRY 19, 21
REFLEX NERVE DISEASES 33
RELAXANT HERB 48, 67
RESTORATIVE 47
RHEUMATISM 51, 68

RICHARDS, WILLARD 71
RINGWORM 64
ROSE HIPS 19, 20, 21
ROSEMARY 58, 59, 60
RUNNING SORES 63

SAFFRON 19, 50, 58, 63, 75
SAGE 59, 60
SALAD DRESSING 56
SALMONELLA 23
SARSAPARILLA 64
SASSAFRAS 64
SAVORY 59, 60
SCARLET FEVER 51
SCULLCAP 69, 82
SECOBARBITAL (SECONAL) 12
SEDATIVE 68
SENNA 24
SENSORY NERVES 69
SESAME SEEDS 58
SHAMPOO 58
SINUSES 20
SKIN CANCER 63, 64
SKIN CARE 61
SKIN DISORDERS 39, 64
SLEEP 67
SLIPPERY ELM 64
SOAP 54
SORREL 24
SOUP BROTH 59
SORE THROAT 39, 58
SPASMS 29, 67, 69
SPICES, ON VEGETABLES 59
SPROUTS 27
SQUASH 60
SQUAW ROOT 29
STEROIDS 45, 53
STIFFNESS 50
STIMULANT HERB 47
STOMACH PROBLEMS 39, 59, 68
STUPOR 67, 68
SUCROSE 33
SUGAR 45, 81; AND DIABETES 33ff
SUNFLOWER SEEDS 58
SUNTANNING 65

"SURVIVAL" (POEM) 13
TANSY 24
TARRAGON 59, 60
TESTOSTERONE 32
THOMSON, SAMUEL 48, 71
THYME 59, 60
THYROID GLAND 38, 67
TOMATOES 60
TONSILS 41
TOOTH DECAY 20
TOXEMIA (PREGNANCY) 20
TRANQUILIZERS 68, 69, 77
TRICHINOSIS 23
TUBERCULOSIS 47
TWITCHING MUSCLES 69

ULCERS 64
UPSET 68, 69
URIC ACID 51, 63
URINARY PROBLEMS 36

VALERIAN 69, 82
VARICOSE ULCERS 64
VEGETABLE, WITH HERBS AND SPICES 59
VERVAIN 63
VIOLET
VITAMINS (HERB SOURCES)
  A 19
  B Complex 82
  B1 19
  B2 19
  B6 19; Deficiencies 3, 20
  B12 20
  C 20, 37,
  D 20
  E 21
VOMITING 20, 67

WARTS 64
WATER RETENTION 20
WATERCRESS 20, 21, 22
"WHERE THERE'S A WILL" (POEM) 83
"WHETHER OR NOT" (POEM) 8

WHOOPING COUGH 33
WINTERGREEN 24, 63
WOOD BETONY 82
"WORK AND GROWTH" (POEM) 75
WORMS 22
WOUNDS 63, 64
YALE, JOHN W. 53
YELLOW DOCK 21
YUCCA 53